W9-BNB-454

FUNDAMENTALS OF
PATHOLOGY

MEDICAL COURSE AND STEP 1 REVIEW
2013 EDITION

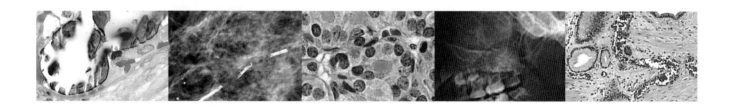

HUSAIN A. SATTAR, MD

Associate Professor of Pathology
Associate Director of Clinical Pathophysiology and Therapeutics
The University of Chicago
Pritzker School of Medicine
Chicago, Illinois

pathoma.com
Chicago • 2013

PATHOMA.COM
Fundamentals of Pathology: Medical Course and Step 1 Review, 2013 Edition

ISBN 978-0-9832246-1-7

Printed in the United States of America.

Copyright © 2013 by Pathoma LLC.

Previous edition copyrighted 2011.

All rights reserved. No part of this publication may be reproduced, distributed, or transmitted in any form, or by any means, electronic or mechanical, including photocopying, recording, or any information storage and retrieval system, without prior permission in writing from the publisher (email: info@pathoma.com).

Disclaimer
Fundamentals of Pathology aims at providing general principles of pathology and its associated disciplines and is not intended as a working guide to patient care, drug administration or treatment. Medicine is a constantly evolving field and changes in practice regularly occur. It is the responsibility of the treating practitioner, relying on independent expertise and knowledge of the patient, to determine the best treatment and method of application for the patient. Neither the publisher nor the author assume any liability for any injury and/or damage to persons or property arising from or related to the material within this publication.

Furthermore, although care has been taken to ensure the accuracy of information present in this publication, the author and publisher make no representations or warranties whatsoever, express or implied, with respect to the completeness, accuracy or currency of the contents of this publication. This publication is not meant to be a substitute for the advice of a physician or other licensed and qualified medical professional. Information presented in this publication may refer to drugs, devices or techniques which are subject to government regulation, and it is the responsibility of the treating practitioner to comply with all applicable laws.

This book is printed on acid-free paper.

Published by Pathoma LLC.
http://www.pathoma.com
info@pathoma.com

Cover and page design by Olaf Nelson, Chinook Design, Inc.
http://www.chinooktype.com

CONTENTS

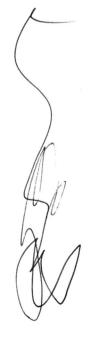

USING THIS BOOK

This work is intended as a review for students during their preclinical years and while preparing for examinations, such as the USMLE™. To this effect, the organization of this book follows that of most primary texts in the field and parallels the syllabus used in pathophysiology courses in medical schools throughout the United States. Ample space is provided for students to make notes during course study and while viewing the online videos that cover each section of the text (www.pathoma.com).

We recommend that students use *Fundamentals of Pathology* during their medical courses, taking notes in the margin as pertinent topics are covered. When exam time comes around, these notes will likely be invaluable.

For examination preparation, we suggest students read the material first, then listen to the online lecture, and then reread the material to develop a solid grasp of each topic. One should not become disheartened if they are not able to retain all the information contained herein. This deceptively slim volume covers a tremendous amount of material, and repetition will be a key aid as you progress in your studies.

An effort has been made to emphasize concepts and principles over random facts, the forest rather than the trees. Attention to the same by the student will provide a deeper, more meaningful understanding of human disease. We must always remind ourselves that ultimately our goal is to learn, to share, and to serve. *Fundamentals of Pathology* was developed with this goal in mind.

Husain A. Sattar, MD
Chicago, Illinois

ACKNOWLEDGMENTS

This work would not have been possible without the support and encouragement of those around me. To begin with, I would like to acknowledge Shaykh Zulfiqar Ahmad, whose clear vision has guided me to horizons I would never have known. My family is to be acknowledged for their limitless sacrifice, in particular the constant encouragement and support of my wife Amina, who has proved through the years to be the wind under my wings. Thomas Krausz, MD and Aliya Husain, MD (both Professors of Pathology at the University of Chicago) deserve particular mention for their valuable advice and guiding vision, both in the development of this book as well as my career. Special thanks to the multiple reviewers at medical centers throughout the country for their critical comments, in particular Mir Basharath Alikhan, MD (Pathology resident, University of Chicago) and Joshua T.B. Williams (Class of 2013, Pritzker School of Medicine, University of Chicago) for their extensive review. Olaf Nelson (Chinook Design, Inc.) is to be commended for his excellent layout and design. Finally, I would be remiss without acknowledging my students, who give meaning to what I do.

TO MY PARENTS AND EACH OF MY TEACHERS—YOUR SACRIFICE
FORMS THE FOUNDATION UPON WHICH OUR WORK IS BUILT

Growth Adaptations, Cellular Injury, and Cell Death

GROWTH ADAPTATIONS

I. BASIC PRINCIPLES
A. An organ is in homeostasis with the physiologic stress placed on it.
B. An increase, decrease, or change in stress on an organ can result in growth adaptations.

II. HYPERPLASIA AND HYPERTROPHY
A. An increase in stress leads to an increase in organ size.
  1. Occurs via an increase in the size (hypertrophy) and/or the number (hyperplasia) of cells
B. Hypertrophy involves gene activation, protein synthesis, and production of organelles.
C. Hyperplasia involves the production of new cells from stem cells.
D. Hyperplasia and hypertrophy generally occur together (e.g., uterus during pregnancy).
  1. Permanent tissues (e.g., cardiac muscle, skeletal muscle, and nerve), however, cannot make new cells and undergo hypertrophy only.
  2. For example, cardiac myocytes undergo hypertrophy, not hyperplasia, in response to systemic hypertension (Fig. 1.1).
E. Pathologic hyperplasia (e.g., endometrial hyperplasia) can progress to dysplasia and, eventually, cancer.
  1. A notable exception is benign prostatic hyperplasia (BPH), which does not increase the risk for prostate cancer.

III. ATROPHY
A. A decrease in stress (e.g., decreased hormonal stimulation, disuse, or decreased nutrients/blood supply) leads to a decrease in organ size (atrophy).
  1. Occurs via a decrease in the size and number of cells.
B. Decrease in cell number occurs via apoptosis.
C. Decrease in cell size occurs via ubiquitin-proteosome degradation of the cytoskeleton and autophagy of cellular components.
  1. In ubiquitin-proteosome degradation, intermediate filaments of the cytoskeleton are "tagged" with ubiquitin and destroyed by proteosomes.
  2. Autophagy of cellular components involves generation of autophagic vacuoles. These vacuoles fuse with lysosomes whose hydrolytic enzymes breakdown cellular components.

IV. METAPLASIA
A. A change in stress on an organ leads to a change in cell type (metaplasia).
  1. Most commonly involves change of one type of surface epithelium (squamous, columnar, or urothelial) to another
  2. Metaplastic cells are better able to handle the new stress.
B. Barrett esophagus is a classic example.

1. Esophagus is normally lined by nonkeratinizing squamous epithelium (suited to handle friction of a food bolus).
2. Acid reflux from the stomach causes metaplasia to nonciliated, mucin-producing columnar cells (better able to handle the stress of acid, Fig. 1.2).

C. Metaplasia occurs via reprogramming of stem cells, which then produce the new cell type.
   1. Metaplasia is reversible, in theory, with removal of the driving stressor.
   2. For example, treatment of gastroesophageal reflux may reverse Barrett esophagus.

D. Under persistent stress, metaplasia can progress to dysplasia and eventually result in cancer.
   1. For example, Barrett esophagus may progress to adenocarcinoma of the esophagus.
   2. A notable exception is apocrine metaplasia of breast, which carries no increased risk for cancer.

E. Vitamin A deficiency can also result in metaplasia.
   1. Vitamin A is necessary for differentiation of specialized epithelial surfaces such as the conjunctiva covering the eye.
   2. In vitamin A deficiency, the thin squamous lining of the conjunctiva undergoes metaplasia into stratified keratinizing squamous epithelium. This change is called keratomalacia (Fig. 1.3).

F. Mesenchymal (connective) tissues can also undergo metaplasia.
   1. A classic example is myositis ossificans in which connective tissue within muscle changes to bone during healing after trauma (Fig. 1.4).

V. DYSPLASIA

A. Disordered cellular growth
B. Most often refers to proliferation of precancerous cells
   1. For example, Cervical intraepithelial neoplasia (CIN) represents dysplasia and is a precursor to cervical cancer.
C. Often arises from longstanding pathologic hyperplasia (e.g., endometrial hyperplasia) or metaplasia (e.g., Barrett esophagus)
D. Dysplasia is reversible, in theory, with alleviation of inciting stress.
   1. If stress persists, dysplasia progresses to carcinoma (irreversible).

VI. APLASIA AND HYPOPLASIA

A. Aplasia is failure of cell production during embryogenesis (e.g., unilateral renal agenesis).
B. Hypoplasia is a decrease in cell production during embryogenesis, resulting in a relatively small organ (e.g., streak ovary in Turner syndrome).

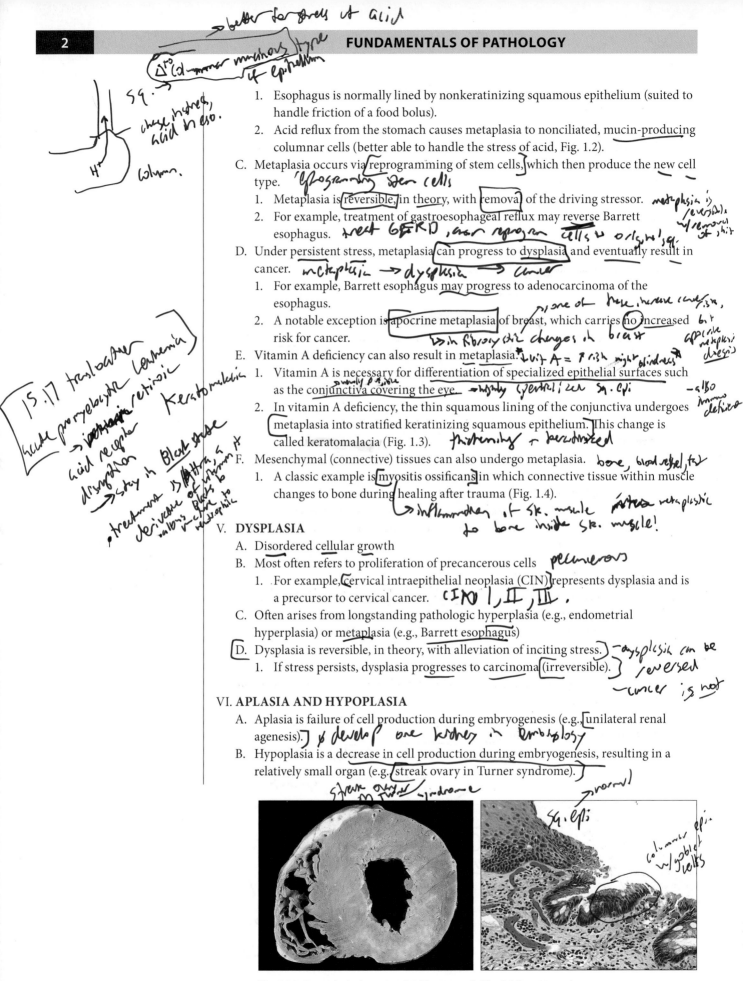

Fig. 1.1 Left ventricular hypertrophy. (Courtesy of Aliya Husain, MD)

Fig. 1.2 Barrett esophagus.

CELLULAR INJURY

I. **BASIC PRINCIPLES**
  A. Cellular injury occurs when a stress exceeds the cell's ability to adapt.
  B. The likelihood of injury depends on the type of stress, its severity, and the type of cell affected.
    1. Neurons are highly susceptible to ischemic injury; whereas, skeletal muscle is relatively more resistant.
    2. Slowly developing ischemia (e.g., renal artery atherosclerosis) results in atrophy; whereas, acute ischemia (e.g., renal artery embolus) results in injury.
  C. Common causes of cellular injury include inflammation, nutritional deficiency or excess, hypoxia, trauma, and genetic mutations.

II. **HYPOXIA**
  A. Low oxygen delivery to tissue; important cause of cellular injury
    1. Oxygen is the final electron acceptor in the electron transport chain of oxidative phosphorylation.
    2. Decreased oxygen impairs oxidative phosphorylation, resulting in decreased ATP production.
    3. Lack of ATP (essential energy source) leads to cellular injury.
  B. Causes of hypoxia include ischemia, hypoxemia, and decreased O_2-carrying capacity of blood.
  C. Ischemia is decreased blood flow through an organ. Arises with
    1. Decreased arterial perfusion (e.g., atherosclerosis)
    2. Decreased venous drainage (e.g., Budd-Chiari syndrome)
    3. Shock—generalized hypotension resulting in poor tissue perfusion
  D. Hypoxemia is a low partial pressure of oxygen in the blood ($Pao_2 < 60$ mm Hg, $Sao_2 < 90\%$). Arises with
    1. High altitude—Decreased barometric pressure results in decreased Pao_2.
    2. Hypoventilation—Increased $Paco_2$ results in decreased Pao_2.
    3. Diffusion defect—Pao_2 not able to push as much O_2 into the blood due to a thicker diffusion barrier (e.g., interstitial pulmonary fibrosis)
    4. V/Q mismatch—Blood bypasses oxygenated lung (circulation problem, e.g., right-to-left shunt), or oxygenated air cannot reach blood (ventilation problem, e.g., atelectasis).
  E. Decreased O_2-carrying capacity arises with hemoglobin (Hb) loss or dysfunction. Examples include
    1. Anemia (decrease in RBC mass)—Pao_2 normal; Sao_2 normal
    2. Carbon monoxide poisoning

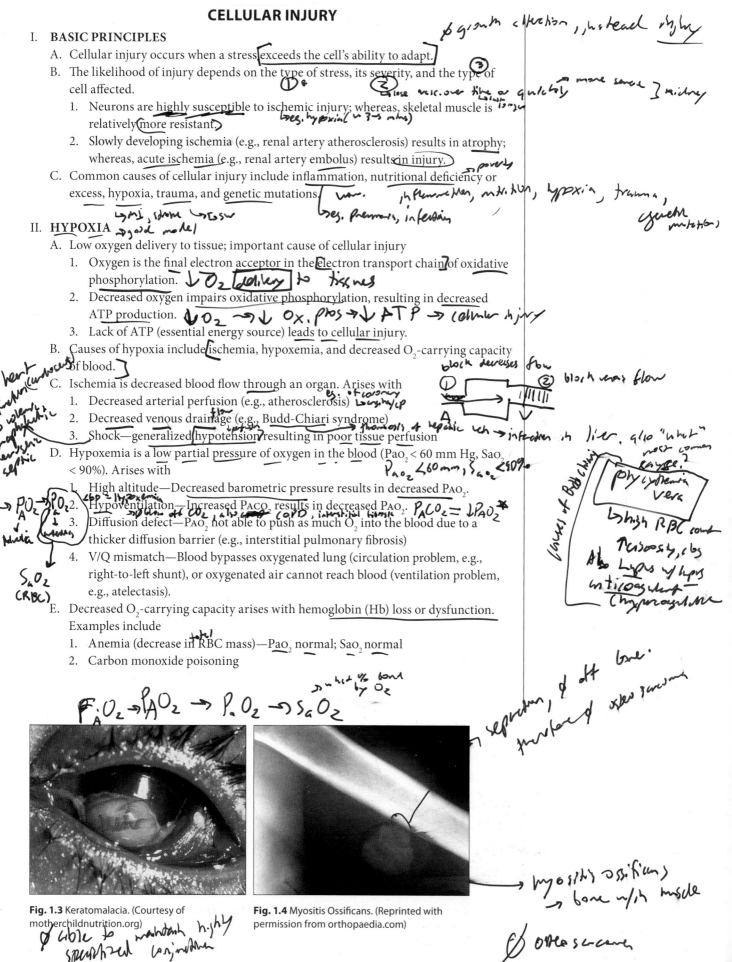

Fig. 1.3 Keratomalacia. (Courtesy of motherchildnutrition.org)

Fig. 1.4 Myositis Ossificans. (Reprinted with permission from orthopaedia.com)

    i. CO binds hemoglobin more avidly than oxygen—Pao_2 normal; Sao_2 decreased

    ii. Exposures include smoke from fires and exhaust from cars or gas heaters.

    iii. Classic finding is cherry-red appearance of skin.

    iv. Early sign of exposure is headache; significant exposure leads to coma and death.

3. Methemoglobinemia

    i. Iron in heme is oxidized to Fe^{3+}, which cannot bind oxygen—Pao_2 normal; Sao_2 decreased

    ii. Seen with oxidant stress (e.g., sulfa and nitrate drugs) or in newborns

    iii. Classic finding is cyanosis with chocolate-colored blood.

    iv. Treatment is intravenous methylene blue, which helps reduce Fe^{3+} back to Fe^{2+} state.

III. REVERSIBLE AND IRREVERSIBLE CELLULAR INJURY

A. Hypoxia impairs oxidative phosphorylation resulting in decreased ATP.

B. Low ATP disrupts key cellular functions including

1. Na^+-K^+ pump, resulting in sodium and water buildup in the cell

2. Ca^{2+} pump, resulting in Ca^{2+} buildup in the cytosol of the cell

3. Aerobic glycolysis, resulting in a switch to anaerobic glycolysis. Lactic acid buildup results in low pH, which denatures proteins and precipitates DNA.

C. The initial phase of injury is reversible. The hallmark of reversible injury is cellular swelling.

1. Cytosol swelling results in loss of microvilli and membrane blebbing.

2. Swelling of the rough endoplasmic reticulum (RER) results in dissociation of ribosomes and decreased protein synthesis.

D. Eventually, the damage becomes irreversible. The hallmark of irreversible injury is membrane damage.

1. Plasma membrane damage results in

    i. Cytosolic enzymes leaking into the serum (e.g., cardiac troponin)

    ii. Additional calcium entering into the cell

2. Mitochondrial membrane damage results in

    i. Loss of the electron transport chain (inner mitochondrial membrane)

    ii. Cytochrome c leaking into cytosol (activates apoptosis)

3. Lysosome membrane damage results in hydrolytic enzymes leaking into the cytosol, which, in turn, are activated by the high intracellular calcium.

E. The end result of irreversible injury is cell death.

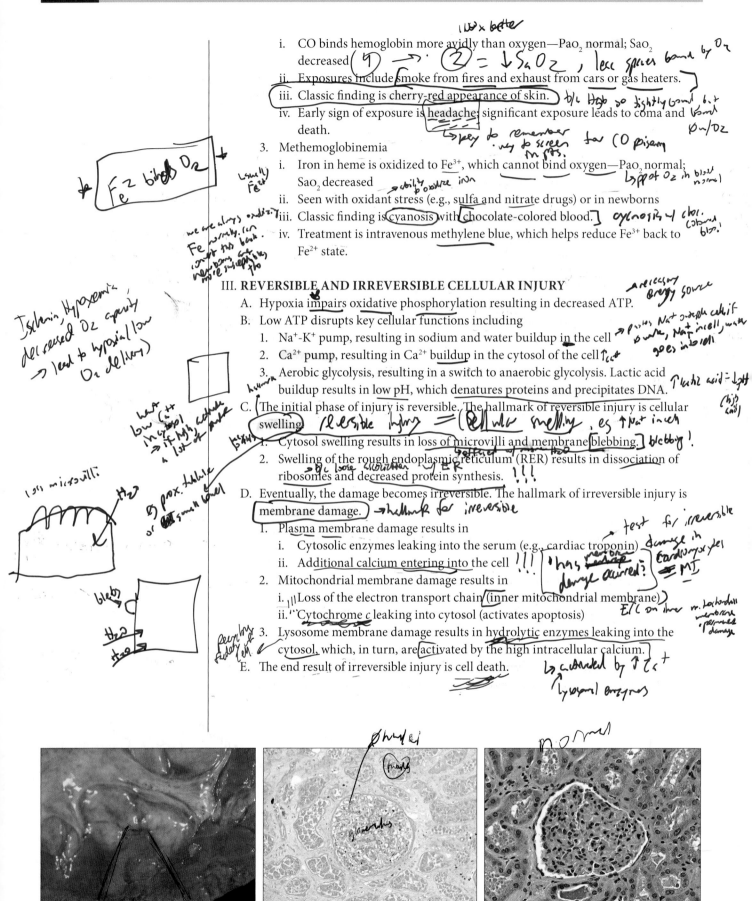

Fig. 1.5 Coagulative necrosis of kidney. **A**, Gross appearance. **B**, Microscopic appearance. **C**, Normal kidney histology for comparison. (A, Courtesy of Aliya Husain, MD)

CELL DEATH

I. **BASIC PRINCIPLES**
   A. The morphologic hallmark of cell death is loss of the nucleus, which occurs via nuclear condensation (pyknosis), fragmentation (karyorrhexis), and dissolution (karyolysis).
   B. The two mechanisms of cell death are necrosis and apoptosis.

II. **NECROSIS**
   A. Death of large groups of cells followed by acute inflammation
   B. Due to some underlying pathologic process; never physiologic
   C. Divided into several types based on gross features

III. **GROSS PATTERNS OF NECROSIS**
   A. Coagulative necrosis
      1. Necrotic tissue that remains firm (Fig. 1.5A); cell shape and organ structure are preserved by coagulation of proteins, but the nucleus disappears (Fig. 1.5B).
      2. Characteristic of ischemic infarction of any organ except the brain
      3. Area of infarcted tissue is often wedge-shaped (pointing to focus of vascular occlusion) and pale.
      4. Red infarction arises if blood re-enters a loosely organized tissue (e.g., pulmonary or testicular infarction, Fig. 1.6).
   B. Liquefactive necrosis
      1. Necrotic tissue that becomes liquefied; enzymatic lysis of cells and protein results in liquefaction.
      2. Characteristic of
         i. Brain infarction—Proteolytic enzymes from microglial cells liquefy the brain.
         ii. Abscess—Proteolytic enzymes from neutrophils liquefy tissue.
         iii. Pancreatitis—Proteolytic enzymes from pancreas liquefy parenchyma.
   C. Gangrenous necrosis
      1. Coagulative necrosis that resembles mummified tissue (dry gangrene, Fig. 1.7)
      2. Characteristic of ischemia of lower limb and GI tract
      3. If superimposed infection of dead tissues occurs, then liquefactive necrosis ensues (wet gangrene).
   D. Caseous necrosis
      1. Soft and friable necrotic tissue with "cottage cheese–like" appearance (Fig. 1.8)
      2. Combination of coagulative and liquefactive necrosis
      3. Characteristic of granulomatous inflammation due to tuberculous or fungal infection

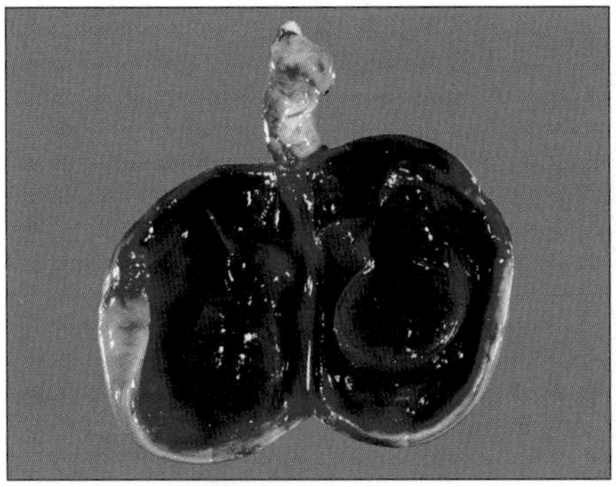

Fig. 1.6 Hemorrhagic infarction of testicle. (Courtesy of humpath.com)

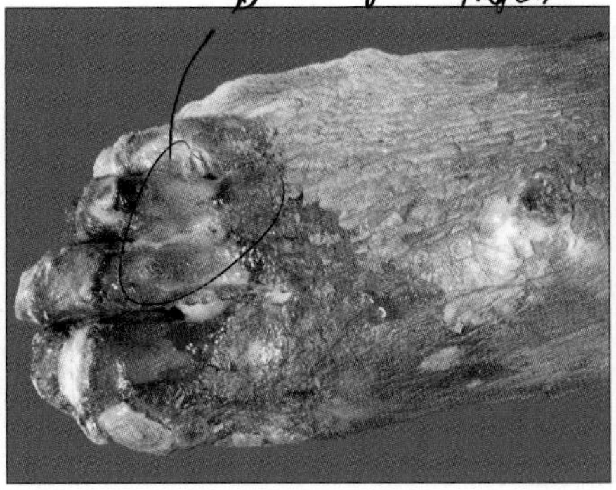

Fig. 1.7 Dry gangrene.

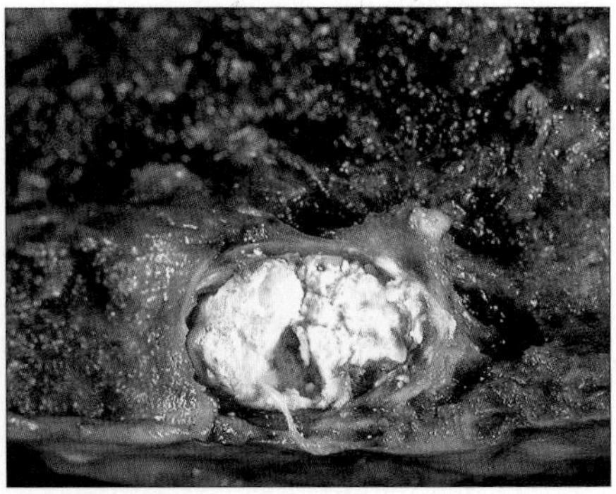

Fig. 1.8 Caseous necrosis of lung. (Courtesy of Yale Rosen, MD)

E. Fat necrosis
1. Necrotic adipose tissue with chalky-white appearance due to deposition of calcium (Fig. 1.9)
2. Characteristic of trauma to fat (e.g., breast) and pancreatitis-mediated damage of peripancreatic fat
3. Fatty acids released by trauma (e.g., to breast) or lipase (e.g., pancreatitis) join with calcium via a process called saponification.
    i. Saponification is an example of dystrophic calcification in which calcium deposits on dead tissues. In dystrophic calcification, the necrotic tissue acts as a nidus for calcification in the setting of *normal* serum calcium and phosphate.
    ii. Metastatic calcification, as opposed to dystrophic calcification, occurs when *high* serum calcium or phosphate levels lead to calcium deposition in normal tissues (e.g., hyperparathyroidism leading to nephrocalcinosis).

F. Fibrinoid necrosis
1. Necrotic damage to blood vessel wall
2. Leaking of proteins (including fibrin) into vessel wall results in bright pink staining of the wall microscopically (Fig. 1.10).
3. Characteristic of malignant hypertension and vasculitis

IV. **APOPTOSIS**
A. Energy (ATP)-dependent, genetically programmed cell death involving single cells or small groups of cells. Examples include
1. Endometrial shedding during menstrual cycle
2. Removal of cells during embryogenesis
3. CD8$^+$ T cell-mediated killing of virally infected cells

B. Morphology
1. Dying cell shrinks, leading cytoplasm to become more eosinophilic (pink, Fig. 1.11).
2. Nucleus condenses and fragments in an organized manner.
3. Apoptotic bodies fall from the cell and are removed by macrophages; apoptosis is not followed by inflammation.

C. Apoptosis is mediated by caspases that activate proteases and endonucleases.
1. Proteases break down the cytoskeleton.
2. Endonucleases break down DNA.

D. Caspases are activated by multiple pathways.
1. Intrinsic mitochondrial pathway
    i. Cellular injury, DNA damage, or decreased hormonal stimulation leads to inactivation of Bcl2.
    ii. Lack of Bcl2 allows cytochrome *c* to leak from the inner mitochondrial matrix into the cytoplasm and activate caspases.

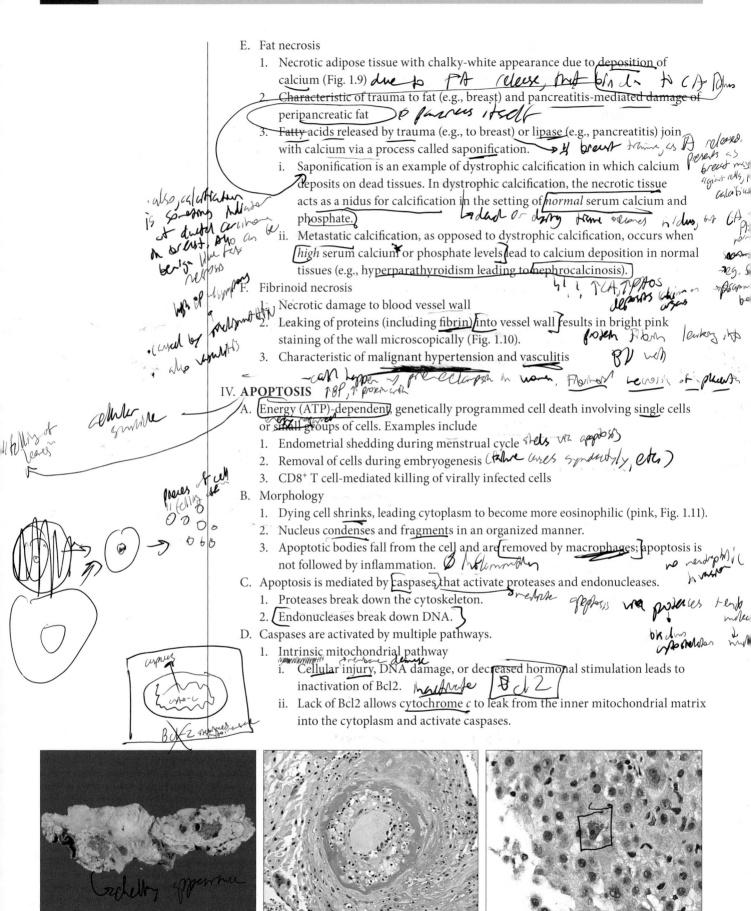

Fig. 1.9 Fat necrosis of peri-pancreatic adipose tissue. (Courtesy of humpath.com)

Fig. 1.10 Fibrinoid necrosis of vessel.

Fig. 1.11 Apoptosis.

2. Extrinsic receptor-ligand pathway
   i. FAS ligand binds FAS death receptor (CD95) on the target cell, activating caspases (e.g., negative selection of thymocytes in thymus).
   ii. Tumor necrosis factor (TNF) binds TNF receptor on the target cell, activating caspases.
3. Cytotoxic $CD8^+$ T cell-mediated pathway
   i. Perforins secreted by $CD8^+$ T cell create pores in membrane of target cell.
   ii. Granzyme from $CD8^+$ T cell enters pores and activates caspases.
   iii. $CD8^+$ T-cell killing of virally infected cells is an example.

FREE RADICAL INJURY

I. **BASIC PRINCIPLES**
   A. Free radicals are chemical species with an unpaired electron in their outer orbit.
   B. Physiologic generation of free radicals occurs during oxidative phosphorylation.
      1. Cytochrome *c* oxidase (complex IV) transfers electrons to oxygen.
      2. Partial reduction of O_2 yields superoxide (O_2^-), hydrogen peroxide (H_2O_2), and hydroxyl radicals ($^{\cdot}OH$).
   C. Pathologic generation of free radicals arises with
      1. Ionizing radiation—water hydrolyzed to hydroxyl free radical
      2. Inflammation—NADPH oxidase generates superoxide ions during oxygen-dependent killing by neutrophils.
      3. Metals (e.g., copper and iron)—Fe^{2+} generates hydroxyl free radicals (Fenton reaction).
      4. Drugs and chemicals—P450 system of liver metabolizes drugs (e.g., acetaminophen), generating free radicals.
   D. Free radicals cause cellular injury via peroxidation of lipids and oxidation of DNA and proteins; DNA damage is implicated in aging and oncogenesis.
   E. Elimination of free radicals occurs via multiple mechanisms.
      1. Antioxidants (e.g., glutathione and vitamins A, C, and E)
      2. Enzymes
         i. Superoxide dismutase (in mitochondria)—Superoxide ($O_2^{\cdot}$) → H_2O_2
         ii. Glutathione peroxidase (in mitochondria)—2GSH + free radical → GS-SG and H_2O
         iii. Catalase (in peroxisomes)—H_2O_2 → O_2 and H_2O
      3. Metal carrier proteins (e.g., transferrin and ceruloplasmin)

II. **EXAMPLES OF FREE RADICAL INJURY**
   A. Carbon tetrachloride (CCl_4)
      1. Organic solvent used in the dry cleaning industry
      2. Converted to CCl_3 free radical by P450 system of hepatocytes
      3. Results in cell injury with swelling of RER; consequently, ribosomes detach, impairing protein synthesis.
      4. Decreased apolipoproteins lead to fatty change in the liver (Fig. 1.12).
   B. Reperfusion injury
      1. Return of blood to ischemic tissue results in production of O_2-derived free radicals, which further damage tissue
      2. Leads to a continued rise in cardiac enzymes (e.g., troponin) after reperfusion of infarcted myocardial tissue

AMYLOIDOSIS

I. **BASIC PRINCIPLES**

    A. Amyloid is a misfolded protein that deposits in the extracellular space, thereby damaging tissues.

    B. Multiple proteins can deposit as amyloid. Shared features include

        1. β-pleated sheet configuration

        2. Congo red staining and apple-green birefringence when viewed microscopically under polarized light (Fig. 1.13)

    C. Deposition can be systemic or localized.

II. **SYSTEMIC AMYLOIDOSIS**

    A. Amyloid deposition in multiple organs; divided into primary and secondary amyloidosis

    B. Primary amyloidosis is systemic deposition of AL amyloid, which is derived from immunoglobulin light chain.

        1. Associated with plasma cell dyscrasias (e.g, multiple myeloma)

    C. Clinical findings of systemic amyloidosis are diverse since almost any tissue can be involved. Classic findings include

        1. SAA is an acute phase reactant that is increased in chronic inflammatory states, malignancy, and Familial Mediterranean fever (FMF).

        2. FMF is due to a dysfunction of neutrophils (autosomal recessive) and occurs in persons of Mediterranean origin.

            i. Presents with episodes of fever and acute serosal inflammation (can mimic appendicitis, arthritis, or myocardial infarction)

            ii. High SAA during attacks deposits as AA amyloid in tissues.

    D. Clinical findings of systemic amyloidosis are diverse since almost any tissue can be involved. Classic findings include

        1. Nephrotic syndrome (kidney is the most common organ involved).

        2. Restrictive cardiomyopathy or arrhythmia

        3. Tongue enlargement, malabsorption, and hepatosplenomegaly

    E. Diagnosis requires tissue biopsy. Abdominal fat pad and rectum are easily accessible biopsy targets.

    F. Damaged organs must be transplanted. Amyloid cannot be removed.

III. **LOCALIZED AMYLOIDOSIS**

    A. Amyloid deposition usually localized to a single organ.

    B. Senile cardiac amyloidosis

        1. Non-mutated serum transthyretin deposits in the heart.

        2. Usually asymptomatic; present in 25% of individuals > 80 years of age

    C. Familial amyloid cardiomyopathy

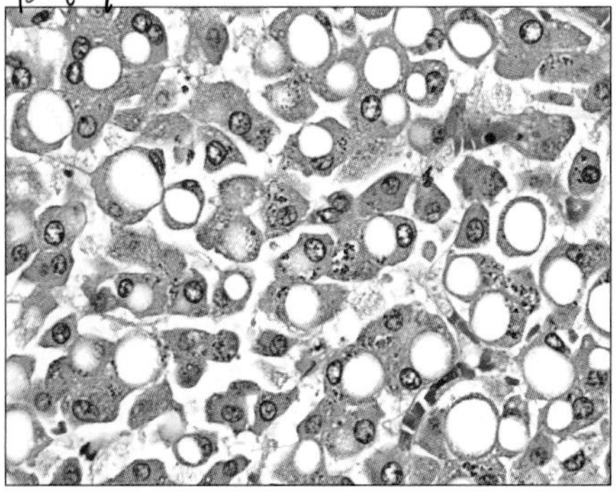

Fig. 1.12 Fatty change of liver.

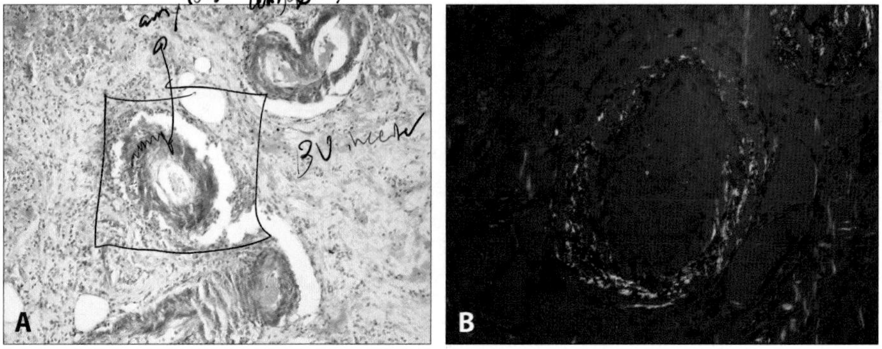

Fig. 1.13 Amyloid. **A**, Congo red. **B**, Apple-green birefringence. (Courtesy of Ed Uthman, MD)

leads to disease

1. Mutated serum transthyretin deposits in the heart leading to restrictive cardiomyopathy.
2. 5% of African Americans carry the mutated gene.

D. Non-insulin-dependent diabetes mellitus (type II) *DM II*
   1. Amylin (derived from insulin) deposits in the islets of the pancreas.

byproduct of ↑ much insulin

Amylin deposits in pancreas

E. Alzheimer disease
   1. Aβ amyloid (derived from β-amyloid precursor protein) deposits in the brain forming amyloid plaques.
   2. Gene for β–APP is present on chromosome 21. Most individuals with Down syndrome (trisomy 21) develop Alzheimer disease by the age of 40 (early-onset).

present on 21, many w/ trisomy 21 get Alzheimer's

F. Dialysis-associated amyloidosis
   1. β2-microglobulin deposits in joints.

B2 microglobulin, in joints, pts on dialysis

filtered out in dialysis

G. Medullary carcinoma of the thyroid → *tumor derived from C-cells*
   1. Calcitonin (produced by tumor cells) deposits within the tumor ('tumor cells in an amyloid background').

MHC I is on nucleated cells & PLTS

B2 MW shown

C-cells produce calcitonin, create amyloid deposits of excess calcitonin.
neuroendocrine protein

histology . "tumor cells in amyloid background"

appear to plasma support MHC I

Dialysis of little B2mg

REMINDER

Thank you for choosing Pathoma for your studies. We strive to provide the highest quality educational materials while keeping affordability in mind. A tremendous amount of time and effort has gone into developing these materials, so we appreciate your legitimate use of this program. It speaks to your integrity as a future physician and the high ethical standards that we all set forth for ourselves when taking the Hippocratic oath. Unauthorized use of Pathoma materials is contrary to the ethical standards of a training physician and is a violation of copyright. Pathoma videos are updated on a regular basis and the most current version, as well as a complete list of errata, can be accessed through your account at Pathoma.com.

Sincerely,

Dr. Sattar, MD

thyroid biopsied by fine needle aspiration

Inflammation, Inflammatory Disorders, and Wound Healing

2

INTRODUCTION

I. INFLAMMATION

A. Allows inflammatory cells, plasma proteins (e.g., complement), and fluid to exit blood vessels and enter the interstitial space

B. Divided into acute and chronic inflammation

ACUTE INFLAMMATION

I. BASIC PRINCIPLES

A. Characterized by the presence of edema and neutrophils in tissue (Fig. 2.1A)

B. Arises in response to infection (to eliminate pathogen) or tissue necrosis (to clear necrotic debris)

C. Immediate response with limited specificity (innate immunity)

II. MEDIATORS OF ACUTE INFLAMMATION

A. Toll-like receptors (TLRs)

1. Present on cells of the innate immune system (e.g., macrophages and dendritic cells)

2. Activated by pathogen-associated molecular patterns (PAMPs) that are commonly shared by microbes

   i. CD14 (a co-receptor for TLR4) on macrophages recognizes lipopoly-saccharide (a PAMP) on the outer membrane of gram-negative bacteria.

3. TLR activation results in upregulation of NF-κB, a nuclear transcription factor that activates immune response genes leading to production of multiple immune mediators.

4. TLRs are also present on cells of adaptive immunity (e.g., lymphocytes) and, hence, play an important role in mediating chronic inflammation.

B. Arachidonic acid (AA) metabolites

1. AA is released from the phospholipid cell membrane by phospholipase A_2 and then acted upon by cyclooxygenase or 5-lipoxygenase.

   i. Cyclooxygenase produces prostaglandins (PG).

      a. PGI_2, PGD_2, and PGE_2 mediate vasodilation and increased vascular permeability.

      b. PGE_2 also mediates pain and fever.

   ii. 5-lipoxygenase produces leukotrienes (LT).

      a. LTB_4 attracts and activates neutrophils.

      b. LTC_4, LTD_4, and LTE_4 (slow reacting substances of anaphylaxis) mediate vasoconstriction, bronchospasm, and increased vascular permeability.

C. Mast cells

1. Widely distributed throughout connective tissue

2. Activated by (1) tissue trauma, (2) complement proteins C3a and C5a, or (3) cross-linking of cell-surface IgE by antigen

       i. Immediate response involves release of preformed histamine granules, which mediate vasodilation of arterioles and increased vascular permeability.

      ii. Delayed response involves production of arachidonic acid metabolites, particularly leukotrienes.

D. Complement

    1. Proinflammatory serum proteins that "complement" inflammation

    2. Circulate as inactive precursors; activation occurs via

      i. Classical pathway—C1 binds IgG or IgM that is bound to antigen.

      ii. Alternative pathway—Microbial products directly activate complement.

      iii. Mannose-binding lectin (MBL) pathway—MBL binds to mannose on microorganisms and activates complement.

    3. All pathways result in production of C3 convertase (mediates C3 → C3a and C3b), which, in turn, produces C5 convertase (mediates C5 → C5a and C5b). C5b complexes with C6-C9 to form the membrane attack complex (MAC).

      i. C3a and C5a (anaphylatoxins)—trigger mast cell degranulation, resulting in histamine-mediated vasodilation and increased vascular permeability

      ii. C5a—chemotactic for neutrophils

      iii. C3b—opsonin for phagocytosis

      iv. MAC—lyses microbes by creating a hole in the cell membrane

E. Hageman factor (Factor XII)

    1. Inactive proinflammatory protein produced in liver

    2. Activated upon exposure to subendothelial or tissue collagen; in turn, activates

      i. Coagulation and fibrinolytic systems

      ii. Complement

      iii. Kinin system—Kinin cleaves high-molecular-weight kininogen (HMWK) to bradykinin, which mediates vasodilation and increased vascular permeability (similar to histamine), as well as pain.

III. **CARDINAL SIGNS OF INFLAMMATION**

A. Redness (rubor) and warmth (calor)

    1. Due to vasodilation, which results in increased blood flow

    2. Occurs via relaxation of arteriolar smooth muscle; key mediators are histamine, prostaglandins, and bradykinin.

B. Swelling (tumor)

    1. Due to leakage of fluid from postcapillary venules into the interstitial space (exudate)

    2. Key mediators are (1) histamine, which causes endothelial cell contraction and (2) tissue damage, resulting in endothelial cell disruption.

C. Pain (dolor)

    1. Bradykinin and PGE_2 sensitize sensory nerve endings.

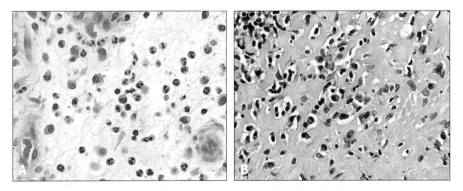

Fig. 2.1 Inflammation. **A,** Acute inflammation with neutrophils. **B,** Chronic inflammation with lymphocytes and plasma cells.

   D. Fever
     1. Pyrogens (e.g., LPS from bacteria) cause macrophages to release IL-1 and TNF, which increase cyclooxygenase activity in perivascular cells of the hypothalamus.
     2. Increased PGE_2 raises temperature set point.

IV. NEUTROPHIL ARRIVAL AND FUNCTION
   A. Step 1—Margination
     1. Vasodilation slows blood flow in postcapillary venules.
     2. Cells marginate from center of flow to the periphery.
   B. Step 2—Rolling
     1. Selectin "speed bumps" are upregulated on endothelial cells.
       i. P-selectin release from Weibel-Palade bodies is mediated by histamine.
       ii. E-selectin is induced by TNF and IL-1.
     2. Selectins bind sialyl Lewis X on leukocytes.
     3. Interaction results in rolling of leukocytes along vessel wall.
   C. Step 3—Adhesion
     1. Cellular adhesion molecules (ICAM and VCAM) are upregulated on endothelium by TNF and IL-1.
     2. Integrins are upregulated on leukocytes by C5a and LTB_4.
     3. Interaction between CAMs and integrins results in firm adhesion of leukocytes to the vessel wall.
     4. Leukocyte adhesion deficiency is most commonly due to an autosomal recessive defect of integrins (CD18 subunit).
       i. Clinical features include delayed separation of the umbilical cord, increased circulating neutrophils (due to impaired adhesion of marginated pool of leukocytes), and recurrent bacterial infections that lack pus formation.
   D. Step 4—Transmigration and Chemotaxis
     1. Leukocytes transmigrate across the endothelium of postcapillary venules and move toward chemical attractants (chemotaxis).
     2. Neutrophils are attracted by bacterial products, IL-8, C5a, and LTB_4.
   E. Step 5—Phagocytosis
     1. Consumption of pathogens or necrotic tissue; phagocytosis is enhanced by opsonins (IgG and C3b).
     2. Pseudopods extend from leukocytes to form phagosomes, which are internalized and merge with lysosomes to produce phagolysosomes.
     3. Chediak-Higashi syndrome is a protein trafficking defect (autosomal recessive) characterized by impaired phagolysosome formation. Clinical features include
       i. Increased risk of pyogenic infections
       ii. Neutropenia (due to intramedullary death of neutrophils)
       iii. Giant granules in leukocytes (due to fusion of granules arising from the Golgi apparatus)
       iv. Defective primary hemostasis (due to abnormal dense granules in platelets)
       v. Albinism
       vi. Peripheral neuropathy
   F. Step 6—Destruction of phagocytosed material
     1. O_2-dependent killing is the most effective mechanism.
     2. HOCl generated by oxidative burst in phagolysosomes destroys phagocytosed microbes.
       i. O_2 is converted to O_2^- by NADPH oxidase (oxidative burst).
       ii. O_2^- is converted to H_2O_2 by superoxide dismutase (SOD).
       iii. H_2O_2 is converted to HOCl (bleach) by myeloperoxidase (MPO).

3. Chronic granulomatous disease (CGD) is characterized by poor O_2-dependent killing.
    i. Due to NADPH oxidase defect (X-linked or autosomal recessive)
    ii. Leads to recurrent infection and granuloma formation with catalase-positive organisms, particularly *Staphylococcus aureus*, *Pseudomonas cepacia*, *Serratia marcescens*, *Nocardia*, and *Aspergillus*
    iii. Nitroblue tetrazolium test is used to screen for CGD. Leukocytes are incubated with NBT dye, which turns blue if NADPH oxidase can convert O_2 to O_2^-, but remains colorless if NADPH oxidase is defective.
4. MPO deficiency results in defective conversion of H_2O_2 to HOCl.
    i. Increased risk for Candida infections; however, most patients are asymptomatic.
    ii. NBT is normal; respiratory burst (O_2 to H_2O_2) is intact.
5. O_2-independent killing is less effective than O_2-dependent killing and occurs via enzymes present in leukocyte secondary granules (e.g., lysozyme in macrophages and major basic protein in eosinophils).
G. Step 7—Resolution
    1. Neutrophils undergo apoptosis and disappear within 24 hours after resolution of the inflammatory stimulus.

V. **MACROPHAGES**
A. Macrophages predominate after neutrophils and peak 2–3 days after inflammation begins.
    1. Derived from monocytes in blood
B. Arrive in tissue via the margination, rolling, adhesion, and transmigration sequence
C. Ingest organisms via phagocytosis (augmented by opsonins) and destroy phagocytosed material using enzymes (e.g., lysozyme) in secondary granules (O_2-independent killing)
D. Manage the next step of the inflammatory process. Outcomes include
    1. Resolution and healing—Anti-inflammatory cytokines (e.g., IL-10 and TGF-β) are produced by macrophages.
    2. Continued acute inflammation—marked by persistent pus formation; IL-8 from macrophages recruits additional neutrophils.
    3. Abscess—acute inflammation surrounded by fibrosis; macrophages mediate fibrosis via fibrogenic growth factors and cytokines.
    4. Chronic inflammation—Macrophages present antigen to activate CD4⁺ helper T cells, which secrete cytokines that promote chronic inflammation.

CHRONIC INFLAMMATION

I. **BASIC PRINCIPLES**
A. Characterized by the presence of lymphocytes and plasma cells in tissue (Fig. 2.1B)
B. Delayed response, but more specific (adaptive immunity) than acute inflammation
C. Stimuli include (1) persistent infection (most common cause); (2) infection with viruses, mycobacteria, parasites, and fungi; (3) autoimmune disease; (4) foreign material; and (5) some cancers.

II. **T LYMPHOCYTES**
A. Produced in bone marrow as progenitor T cells
B. Further develop in the thymus where the T-cell receptor (TCR) undergoes rearrangement and progenitor cells become CD4⁺ helper T cells or CD8⁺ cytotoxic T cells
    1. T cells use TCR complex (TCR and CD3) for antigen surveillance.

     2. TCR complex recognizes antigen presented on MHC molecules.
       i. CD4$^+$ T cells—MHC class II
       ii. CD8$^+$ T cells—MHC class I
     3. Activation of T cells requires (1) binding of antigen/MHC complex and (2) an additional 2nd signal.

C. CD4$^+$ helper T-cell activation
     1. Extracellular antigen (e.g., foreign protein) is phagocytosed, processed, and presented on MHC class II, which is expressed by antigen presenting cells (APCs).
     2. B7 on APC binds CD28 on CD4$^+$ helper T cells providing 2nd activation signal.
     3. Activated CD4$^+$ helper T cells secrete cytokines that "help" inflammation and are divided into two subsets.
       i. T$_H$1 subset secretes IFN-γ (activates macrophage, promotes B-cell class switching from IgM to IgG, promotes T$_H$1 phenotype and inhibits T$_H$2 phenotype).
       ii. T$_H$2 subset secretes IL-4 (facilitates B-cell class switching to IgE), IL-5 (eosinophil chemotaxis and activation, and class switching to IgA), and IL-13 (function similar to IL-4).

D. CD8$^+$ cytotoxic T-cell activation
     1. Intracellular antigen (derived from proteins in the cytoplasm) is processed and presented on MHC class I, which is expressed by all nucleated cells and platelets.
     2. IL-2 from CD4$^+$ T$_H$1 cell provides 2nd activation signal.
     3. Cytotoxic T cells are activated for killing.
     4. Killing occurs via
       i. Secretion of perforin and granzyme; perforin creates pores that allow granzyme to enter the target cell, activating apoptosis.
       ii. Expression of FasL, which binds Fas on target cells, activating apoptosis

III. B LYMPHOCYTES

A. Immature B cells are produced in the bone marrow and undergo immunoglobulin rearrangements to become naïve B cells that express surface IgM and IgD.
B. B-cell activation occurs via
     1. Antigen binding by surface IgM or IgD; results in maturation to IgM- or IgD-secreting plasma cells
     2. B-cell antigen presentation to CD4$^+$ helper T cells via MHC class II.
       i. CD40 receptor on B cell binds CD40L on helper T cell, providing 2nd activation signal.
       ii. Helper T cell then secretes IL-4 and IL-5 (mediate B-cell isotype switching, hypermutation, and maturation to plasma cells).

IV. GRANULOMATOUS INFLAMMATION

A. Subtype of chronic inflammation
B. Characterized by granuloma, which is a collection of epithelioid histiocytes (macrophages with abundant pink cytoplasm), usually surrounded by giant cells and a rim of lymphocytes
C. Divided into noncaseating and caseating subtypes
     1. Noncaseating granulomas lack central necrosis (Fig. 2.2A). Common etiologies include reaction to foreign material, sarcoidosis, beryllium exposure, Crohn disease, and cat scratch disease.
     2. Caseating granulomas exhibit central necrosis and are characteristic of tuberculosis and fungal infections (Fig. 2.2B).
D. Steps involved in granuloma formation

1. Macrophages process and present antigen via MHC class II to CD4⁺ helper T cells.
2. Interaction leads macrophages to secrete IL-12, inducing CD4⁺ helper T cells to differentiate into T_H1 subtype.
3. T_H1 cells secrete IFN-γ, which converts macrophages to epithelioid histiocytes and giant cells.

PRIMARY IMMUNODEFICIENCY

I. **DIGEORGE SYNDROME**
  A. Developmental failure of the third and fourth pharyngeal pouches
     1. Due to 22q11 microdeletion
  B. Presents with T-cell deficiency (lack of thymus); hypocalcemia (lack of parathyroids); and abnormalities of heart, great vessels, and face

II. **SEVERE COMBINED IMMUNODEFICIENCY (SCID)**
  A. Defective cell-mediated and humoral immunity
  B. Etiologies include
     1. Cytokine receptor defects—Cytokine signaling is necessary for proliferation and maturation of B and T cells.
     2. Adenosine deaminase (ADA) deficiency—ADA is necessary to deaminate adenosine and deoxyadenosine for excretion as waste products; buildup of adenosine and deoxyadenosine is toxic to lymphocytes.
     3. MHC class II deficiency—MHC class II is necessary for CD4⁺ helper T cell activation and cytokine production.
  C. Characterized by susceptibility to fungal, viral, bacterial, and protozoal infections, including opportunistic infections and live vaccines
  D. Treatment is sterile isolation ('bubble baby') and stem cell transplantation.

III. **X-LINKED AGAMMAGLOBULINEMIA**
  A. Complete lack of immunoglobulin due to disordered B-cell maturation
     1. Pre- and pro-B cells cannot mature.
  B. Due to mutated Bruton tyrosine kinase; X-linked
  C. Presents after 6 months of life with recurrent bacterial, enterovirus (e.g., polio and coxsackievirus), and *Giardia lamblia* infections; maternal antibodies present during the first 6 months of life are protective.
  D. Live vaccines (e.g., polio) must be avoided.

IV. **COMMON VARIABLE IMMUNODEFICIENCY (CVID)**
  A. Low immunoglobulin due to B-cell or helper T-cell defects

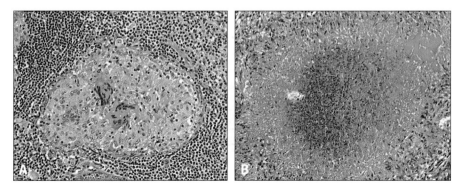

Fig. 2.2 Granuloma. **A**, Noncaseating. **B**, Caseating.

B. Increased risk for bacterial, enterovirus, and *Giardia lamblia* infections, usually in late childhood

C. Increased risk for autoimmune disease and lymphoma

V. IgA DEFICIENCY

A. Low serum and mucosal IgA; most common immunoglobulin deficiency

B. Increased risk for mucosal infection, especially viral; however, most patients are asymptomatic.

VI. HYPER-IgM SYNDROME

A. Characterized by elevated IgM

B. Due to mutated CD40L (on helper T cells) or CD40 receptor (on B cells)
   1. Second signal cannot be delivered to helper T cells during B-cell activation.
   2. Consequently, cytokines necessary for immunoglobulin class switching are not produced.

C. Low IgA, IgG, and IgE result in recurrent pyogenic infections (due to poor opsonization), especially at mucosal sites.

VII. WISKOTT-ALDRICH SYNDROME

A. Characterized by thrombocytopenia, eczema, and recurrent infections (defective humoral and cellular immunity); bleeding is a major cause of death

B. Due to mutation in the WASP gene; X-linked

VIII. COMPLEMENT DEFICIENCIES

A. C5-C9 deficiencies—increased risk for *Neisseria* infection (*N gonorrhoeae* and *N meningitidis*)

B. C1 inhibitor deficiency—results in hereditary angioedema, which is characterized by edema of the skin (especially periorbital, Fig. 2.3) and mucosal surfaces

AUTOIMMUNE DISORDERS

I. BASIC PRINCIPLES

A. Characterized by immune-mediated damage of tissues
   1. 1% prevalence in the US

B. Involves loss of self-tolerance
   1. Self-reactive lymphocytes are regularly generated but undergo apoptosis (negative selection) in the thymus (T cells) or bone marrow (B cells) or become anergic (due to recognition of antigen in peripheral lymphoid tissues with no 2nd signal).

C. More common in women; classically affects women of childbearing age

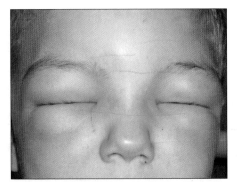

Fig. 2.3 Angioedema. (Courtesy of James Heilman, MD, Wikipedia)

D. Etiology is likely an environmental trigger in genetically susceptible individuals (increased incidence in twins and associated with certain HLA subtypes).

II. **SYSTEMIC LUPUS ERYTHEMATOSUS**
   A. Systemic autoimmune disease
      1. Antibodies against the host damage multiple tissues via type II (cytotoxic) and type III (antigen-antibody complex) hypersensitivity.
      2. More common in women, especially African American females
   B. Clinical features include
      1. Fever and weight loss
      2. Malar 'butterfly' rash (Fig. 2.4), especially upon exposure to sunlight
      3. Arthritis
      4. Pleuritis and pericarditis (involvement of serosal surfaces)
      5. CNS psychosis
      6. Renal damage—Diffuse proliferative glomerulonephritis is the most common injury, though other patterns of injury also occur.
      7. Endocarditis, myocarditis, or pericarditis (can affect any layer of the heart)
         i. Libman-Sacks endocarditis is a classic finding and is characterized by small, sterile deposits on both sides of the mitral valve.
      8. Anemia, thrombocytopenia, or leukopenia (due to autoantibodies against cell surface proteins)
      9. Renal failure and infection are common causes of death.
   C. Characterized by antinuclear antibody (ANA; sensitive, but not specific) and anti-dsDNA antibodies (highly specific)
   D. Antihistone antibody is characteristic of drug-induced SLE.
      1. Hydralazine, procainamide, and isoniazid are common causes.
      2. Removal of drug usually results in remission.
   E. Antiphospholipid antibody syndrome is associated with SLE (30% of cases).
      1. Characterized by autoantibody against proteins bound to phospholipids.
      2. Anticardiolipin and lupus anticoagulant are the most common antibodies.
         i. Lead to false-positive syphilis test and falsely-elevated PTT lab studies, respectively
      3. Results in arterial and venous thrombosis including deep venous thrombosis, hepatic vein thrombosis, placental thrombosis (recurrent pregnancy loss), and stroke
      4. Requires lifelong anticoagulation

III. **SJÖGREN SYNDROME**
   A. Autoimmune destruction of lacrimal and salivary glands
      1. Lymphocyte-mediated damage (type IV hypersensitivity) with fibrosis

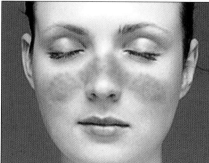

Fig. 2.4 Malar 'butterfly' rash, SLE.

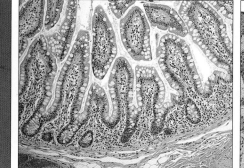

Fig. 2.5 Intestinal crypts.

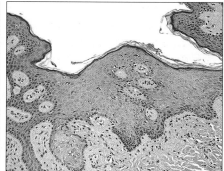

Fig. 2.6 Basal layer of skin.

B. Classically presents as dry eyes (keratoconjunctivitis), dry mouth (xerostomia), and recurrent dental caries in an older woman (50–60 years)—"Can't chew a cracker, dirt in my eyes"

C. Characterized by ANA and anti-ribonucleoprotein antibodies (anti-SS-A/Ro and anti-SS-B/La)

D. Often associated with other autoimmune diseases, especially rheumatoid arthritis

E. Increased risk for B-cell (marginal zone) lymphoma, which presents as unilateral enlargement of the parotid gland late in disease course

IV. SCLERODERMA

A. Autoimmune disease characterized by activation of fibroblasts and deposition of collagen (fibrosis)

B. Divided into localized scleroderma and systemic sclerosis

C. Localized scleroderma involves skin only.
1. Most common subtype is called morphea.
2. Highly associated with antibodies to DNA topoisomerase II

D. Systemic sclerosis involves both skin and visceral organs and is divided into limited and diffuse types.
1. Limited type involves limited areas of skin (mostly hands, face, and neck) with late visceral involvement.
   i. Prototype is CREST syndrome: **C**alcinosis/anti-**C**entromere antibodies, **R**aynaud phenomenon, **E**sophageal dysmotility, **S**clerodactyly, and **T**elangiectasias of the skin.
2. Diffuse type diffusely involves skin and can involve any visceral organ; GI tract, lungs, and kidneys are commonly involved.

V. MIXED CONNECTIVE TISSUE DISEASE

A. Autoimmune-mediated tissue damage with mixed features of SLE, systemic sclerosis, and polymyositis

B. Characterized by serum antibodies against U1 ribonucleoprotein

WOUND HEALING

I. BASIC PRINCIPLES

A. Healing is initiated when inflammation begins.

B. Occurs via a combination of regeneration and repair

II. REGENERATION

A. Replacement of damaged tissue with native tissue; dependent on regenerative capacity of tissue

B. Tissues are divided into three types based on regenerative capacity: labile, stable, and permanent.

C. Labile tissues possess stem cells that continuously cycle to regenerate the tissue.
1. Small and large bowel (stem cells in mucosal crypts, Fig. 2.5)
2. Skin (stem cells in basal layer, Fig. 2.6)
3. Bone marrow (hematopoietic stem cells)

D. Stable tissues are comprised of cells that are quiescent (G_0), but can reenter the cell cycle to regenerate tissue when necessary.
1. Classic example is regeneration of liver by compensatory hyperplasia after partial resection. Each hepatocyte produces additional cells and then reenters quiescence.

E. Permanent tissues lack significant regenerative potential (e.g., myocardium, skeletal muscle, and neurons).

III. **REPAIR**
   A. Replacement of damaged tissue with fibrous scar
   B. Occurs when regenerative stem cells are lost (e.g., deep skin cut) or when a tissue lacks regenerative capacity (e.g., healing after a myocardial infarction, Fig. 2.7)
   C. Granulation tissue formation is the initial phase of repair (Fig. 2.8).
      1. Consists of fibroblasts (deposit type III collagen), capillaries (provide nutrients), and myofibroblasts (contract wound)
   D. Eventually results in scar formation, in which type III collagen is replaced with type I collagen
      1. Type III collagen is pliable and present in granulation tissue, embryonic tissue, uterus, and keloids.
      2. Type I collagen has high tensile strength and is present in skin, bone, tendons, and most organs.
      3. Collagenase removes type III collagen and requires zinc as a cofactor.

IV. **MECHANISMS OF TISSUE REGENERATION AND REPAIR**
   A. Mediated by paracrine signaling via growth factors (e.g., macrophages secrete growth factors that target fibroblasts)
   B. Interaction of growth factors with receptors (e.g., epidermal growth factor with growth factor receptor) results in gene expression and cellular growth.
   C. Examples of mediators include
      1. TGF-α—epithelial and fibroblast growth factor
      2. TGF-β—important fibroblast growth factor; also inhibits inflammation
      3. Platelet-derived growth factor—growth factor for endothelium, smooth muscle, and fibroblasts
      4. Fibroblast growth factor—important for angiogenesis; also mediates skeletal development
      5. Vascular endothelial growth factor (VEGF)—important for angiogenesis

V. **NORMAL AND ABERRANT WOUND HEALING**
   A. Cutaneous healing occurs via primary or secondary intention.
      1. Primary intention—Wound edges are brought together (e.g., suturing of a surgical incision); leads to minimal scar formation
      2. Secondary intention—Edges are not approximated. Granulation tissue fills the defect; myofibroblasts then contract the wound, forming a scar.
   B. Delayed wound healing occurs in
      1. Infection (most common cause; *S aureus* is the most common offender)
      2. Vitamin C, copper, or zinc deficiency

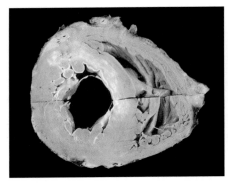

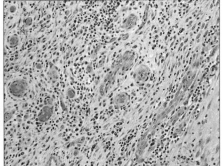

Fig. 2.7 Myocardial scarring. (Courtesy of Aliya Husain, MD)

Fig. 2.8 Granulation tissue.

      i.   Vitamin C is an important cofactor in the hydroxylation of proline and lysine procollagen residues; hydroxylation is necessary for eventual collagen cross-linking.

     ii.   Copper is a cofactor for lysyl oxidase, which cross-links lysine and hydroxylysine to form stable collagen.

   iii.   Zinc is a cofactor for collagenase, which replaces the type III collagen of granulation tissue with stronger type I collagen.

   3. Other causes include foreign body, ischemia, diabetes, and malnutrition.

C. Dehiscence is rupture of a wound; most commonly seen after abdominal surgery

D. Hypertrophic scar is excess production of scar tissue that is localized to the wound (Fig. 2.9).

E. Keloid is excess production of scar tissue that is out of proportion to the wound (Fig. 2.10).

   1. Characterized by excess type III collagen

   2. Genetic predisposition (more common in African Americans)

   3. Classically affects earlobes, face, and upper extremities

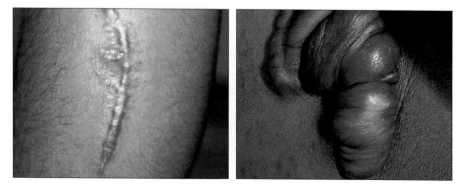

Fig. 2.9 Hypertrophic scar. (Reprinted with permission, http://emedicine.medscape.com/article/1128404-overview)

Fig. 2.10 Keloid.

Principles of Neoplasia

NEOPLASIA

I. **BASIC PRINCIPLES**
   A. Neoplasia is new tissue growth that is unregulated, irreversible, and monoclonal; these features distinguish it from hyperplasia and repair.
   B. Monoclonal means that the neoplastic cells are derived from a single mother cell.
   C. Clonality was historically determined by glucose-6-phosphate dehydrogenase (G6PD) enzyme isoforms.
      1. Multiple isoforms (e.g., $G6PD_A$, $G6PD_B$, and $G6PD_C$) exist; only one isoform is inherited from each parent.
      2. In females, one isoform is randomly inactivated in each cell by lyonization (G6PD is present on the X chromosome).
      3. Normal ratio of active isoforms in cells of any tissue is 1:1 (e.g., 50% of cells have $G6PD_A$, and 50% of cells have $G6PD_B$).
      4. 1:1 ratio is maintained in hyperplasia, which is polyclonal (cells are derived from multiple cells).
      5. Only one isoform is present in neoplasia, which is monoclonal.
      6. Clonality can also be determined by androgen receptor isoforms, which are also present on the X chromosome.
   D. Clonality of B lymphocytes is determined by immunoglobulin (Ig) light chain phenotype.
      1. Ig is comprised of heavy and light chains.
      2. Each B cell expresses light chain that is either kappa or lambda.
      3. Normal kappa to lambda light chain ratio is 3:1.
      4. This ratio is maintained in hyperplasia, which is polyclonal.
      5. Ratio increases to > 6:1 or is inverted (e.g., kappa to lambda ratio = 1:3) in lymphoma, which is monoclonal.
   E. Neoplastic tumors are benign or malignant.
      1. Benign tumors remain localized and do not metastasize.
      2. Malignant tumors (cancer) invade locally and have the potential to metastasize.
   F. Tumor nomenclature is based on lineage of differentiation (type of tissue produced) and whether the tumor is benign or malignant (Table 3.1).

Table 3.1: Examples of Tumor Nomenclature

LINEAGE OF DIFFERENTIATION	BENIGN	MALIGNANT (CANCER)
Epithelium	Adenoma	Adenocarcinoma
	Papilloma	Papillary carcinoma
Mesenchyme	Lipoma	Liposarcoma
Lymphocyte	(Does not exist)	Lymphoma/Leukemia
Melanocyte	Nevus (mole)	Melanoma

II. **EPIDEMIOLOGY**
   A. Cancer is the 2nd leading cause of death in both adults and children.
      1. The leading causes of death in adults are (1) cardiovascular disease, (2) cancer, and (3) chronic respiratory disease.
      2. The leading causes of death in children are (1) accidents, (2) cancer, and (3) congenital defects.
   B. The most common cancers by incidence in adults are (1) breast/prostate, (2) lung, and (3) colorectal.
   C. The most common causes of cancer mortality in adults are (1) lung, (2) breast/prostate, and (3) colorectal.

III. **ROLE OF SCREENING**
   A. Cancer begins as a single mutated cell.
   B. Approximately 30 divisions occur before the earliest clinical symptoms arise.
   C. Each division (doubling time) results in increased mutations.
      1. Cancers that do not produce symptoms until late in disease will have undergone additional divisions and, hence, additional mutations.
      2. Cancers that are detected late tend to have a poor prognosis.
   D. Goal of screening is to catch dysplasia (precancerous change) before it becomes carcinoma or carcinoma before clinical symptoms arise.
   E. Common screening methods include
      1. Pap smear—detects cervical dysplasia (CIN) before it becomes carcinoma
      2. Mammography—detects in situ breast cancer (e.g., DCIS) before it invades or invasive carcinoma before it becomes clinically palpable
      3. Prostate specific antigen (PSA) and digital rectal exam—detects prostate carcinoma before it spreads
      4. Hemoccult test (for occult blood in stool) and colonoscopy—detect colonic adenoma before it becomes colonic carcinoma or carcinoma before it spreads

CARCINOGENESIS

I. **BASIC PRINCIPLES**
   A. Cancer formation is initiated by damage to DNA of stem cells. The damage overcomes DNA repair mechanisms, but is not lethal.
      1. Carcinogens are agents that damage DNA, increasing the risk for cancer. Important carcinogens include chemicals, oncogenic viruses, and radiation (Table 3.2).
   B. DNA mutations eventually disrupt key regulatory systems, allowing for tumor promotion (growth) and progression (spread).
      1. Disrupted systems include proto-oncogenes, tumor suppressor genes, and regulators of apoptosis.

II. **ONCOGENES**
   A. Proto-oncogenes are essential for cell growth and differentiation; mutations of proto-oncogenes form oncogenes that lead to unregulated cellular growth.
   B. Categories of oncogenes include growth factors, growth factor receptors, signal transducers, nuclear regulators, and cell cycle regulators (Table 3.3).
      1. Growth factors induce cellular growth (e.g., *PDGFB* in astrocytoma).
      2. Growth factor receptors mediate signals from growth factors (e.g., *ERBB2* [*HER2/neu*] in breast cancer).
      3. Signal transducers relay receptor activation to the nucleus (e.g., ras).
         i. Ras is associated with growth factor receptors in an inactive GDP-bound state.

Table 3.2: Important Carcinogens and Associated Cancers

CARCINOGENIC AGENT	ASSOCIATED CANCER	COMMENTS
CHEMICALS		
Aflatoxins	Hepatocellular carcinoma	Derived from *Aspergillus,* which can contaminate stored rice and grains
Alkylating agents	Leukemia/lymphoma	Side effect of chemotherapy
Alcohol	Squamous cell carcinoma of oropharynx and upper esophagus, and hepatocellular carcinoma	
Arsenic	Squamous cell carcinoma of skin, lung cancer, and angiosarcoma of liver	Arsenic is present in cigarette smoke.
Asbestos	Lung carcinoma and mesothelioma	Exposure to asbestos is more likely to lead to lung cancer than mesothelioma.
Cigarette smoke	Carcinoma of oropharynx, esophagus, lung, kidney, bladder, and pancreas	Most common carcinogen worldwide; polycyclic hydrocarbons are particularly carcinogenic.
Nitrosamines	Stomach carcinoma	Found in smoked foods; responsible for high rate of stomach carcinoma in Japan
Naphthylamine	Urothelial carcinoma of bladder	Derived from cigarette smoke
Vinyl chloride	Angiosarcoma of liver	Occupational exposure; used to make polyvinyl chloride (PVC) for use in pipes
Nickel, chromium, beryllium, or silica	Lung carcinoma	Occupational exposure
ONCOGENIC VIRUSES		
EBV	Nasopharyngeal carcinoma, Burkitt lymphoma, and CNS lymphoma in AIDS	
HHV-8	Kaposi sarcoma	
HBV and HCV	Hepatocellular carcinoma	
HTLV-1	Adult T-cell leukemia/lymphoma	
High-risk HPV (e.g., subtypes 16, 18, 31, 33)	Squamous cell carcinoma of vulva, vagina, anus, and cervix; adenocarcinoma of cervix	
RADIATION		
Ionizing (nuclear reactor accidents and radiotherapy)	AML, CML, and papillary carcinoma of the thyroid	Generates hydroxyl free radicals
Nonionizing (UVB sunlight is most common source)	Basal cell carcinoma, squamous cell carcinoma, and melanoma of skin	Results in formation of pyrimidine dimers in DNA, which are normally excised by restriction endonuclease

  ii. Receptor binding causes GDP to be replaced with GTP, activating ras.

  iii. Activated ras sends growth signals to the nucleus.

  iv. Ras inactivates itself by cleaving GTP to GDP; this is augmented by GTPase activating protein.

  v. Mutated ras inhibits the activity of GTPase activating protein. This prolongs the activated state of ras, resulting in increased growth signals.

 4. Cell cycle regulators mediate progression through the cell cycle (e.g., cyclin and cyclin-dependent kinase).

  i. Cyclins and cyclin-dependent kinases (CDKs) form a complex which phosphorylates proteins that drive the cell through the cell cycle.

  ii. For example, the cyclinD/CDK4 complex phosphorylates the retinoblastoma protein, which promotes progression through the G_1/S checkpoint.

III. TUMOR SUPPRESSOR GENES

 A. Regulate cell growth and, hence, decrease ("suppress") the risk of tumor formation; p53 and Rb (retinoblastoma) are classic examples.

 B. p53 regulates progression of the cell cycle from G_1 to S phase.

  1. In response to DNA damage, p53 slows the cell cycle and upregulates DNA repair enzymes.

Table 3.3: Important Oncogenes and Associated Tumors

	FUNCTION	MECHANISM	ASSOCIATED TUMOR
GROWTH FACTOR			
PDGFB	Platelet-derived growth factor	Overexpression, autocrine loop	Astrocytoma
GROWTH FACTOR RECEPTORS			
ERBB2 [HER2/neu]	Epidermal growth factor receptor	Amplification	Subset of breast carcinomas
RET	Neural growth factor receptor	Point mutation	MEN 2A, MEN 2B and sporadic medullary carcinoma of thyroid
KIT	Stem cell growth factor receptor	Point mutation	Gastrointestinal stromal tumor
SIGNAL TRANSDUCERS			
RAS gene family	GTP-binding protein	Point mutation	Carcinomas, melanoma, and lymphoma
ABL	Tyrosine kinase	t(9;22) with BCR	CML and some types of ALL
NUCLEAR REGULATORS			
c-MYC	Transcription factor	t(8;14) involving IgH	Burkitt lymphoma
N-MYC	Transcription factor	Amplification	Neuroblastoma
L-MYC	Transcription factor	Amplification	Lung carcinoma (small cell)
CELL CYCLE REGULATORS			
CCND1 (cyclin D1)	Cyclin	t(11;14) involving IgH	Mantle cell lymphoma
CDK4	Cyclin-dependent kinase	Amplification	Melanoma

2. If DNA repair is not possible, p53 induces apoptosis.
   i. p53 upregulates BAX, which disrupts Bcl2.
   ii. Cytochrome *c* leaks from the mitochondria activating apoptosis.
3. Both copies of the p53 gene must be knocked out for tumor formation (Knudson two-hit hypothesis).
   i. Loss is seen in > 50% of cancers.
   ii. Germline mutation results in Li-Fraumeni syndrome (2nd hit is somatic), characterized by the propensity to develop multiple types of carcinomas and sarcomas.
C. Rb also regulates progression from G_1 to S phase.
1. Rb "holds" the E2F transcription factor, which is necessary for transition to the S phase.
2. E2F is released when *RB* is phosphorylated by the cyclinD/cyclin-dependent kinase 4 (CDK4) complex.
3. Rb mutation results in constitutively free E2F, allowing progression through the cell cycle and uncontrolled growth of cells.
4. Both copies of Rb gene must be knocked out for tumor formation (Knudson two-hit hypothesis).
   i. Sporadic mutation (both hits are somatic) is characterized by unilateral retinoblastoma (Fig. 3.1).
   ii. Germline mutation results in familial retinoblastoma (2nd hit is somatic), characterized by bilateral retinoblastoma and osteosarcoma.

IV. REGULATORS OF APOPTOSIS
A. Prevent apoptosis in normal cells, but promote apoptosis in mutated cells whose DNA cannot be repaired (e.g., Bcl2)
1. Bcl2 normally stabilizes the mitochondrial membrane, blocking release of cytochrome *c*.
2. Disruption of Bcl2 allows cytochrome *c* to leave the mitochondria and activate apoptosis.
B. Bcl2 is overexpressed in follicular lymphoma.
1. t(14;18) moves Bcl2 (chromosome 18) to the Ig heavy chain locus (chromosome 14), resulting in increased Bcl2.
2. Mitochondrial membrane is further stabilized, prohibiting apoptosis.
3. B cells that would normally undergo apoptosis during somatic hypermutation in the lymph node germinal center accumulate, leading to lymphoma.

V. OTHER IMPORTANT FEATURES OF TUMOR DEVELOPMENT
A. Telomerase is necessary for cell immortality.

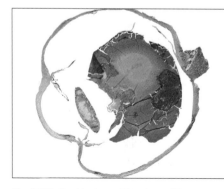

Fig. 3.1 Retinoblastoma. (Courtesy of Jerome Taxy, MD)

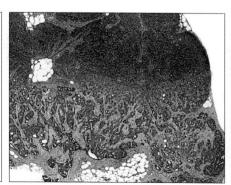

Fig. 3.2 Carcinoma involving lymph node.

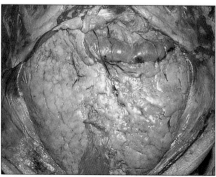

Fig. 3.3 Seeding of the omentum by carcinoma. (Courtesy of Jerome Taxy, MD)

1. Normally, telomeres shorten with serial cell divisions, eventually resulting in cellular senescence.
2. Cancers often have upregulated telomerase, which preserves telomeres.
B. Angiogenesis (production of new blood vessels) is necessary for tumor survival and growth.
   1. FGF and VEGF (angiogenic factors) are commonly produced by tumor cells.
C. Avoiding immune surveillance is necessary for tumor survival.
   1. Mutations often result in production of abnormal proteins, which are expressed on MHC class I.
   2. CD8+ T cells detect and destroy such mutated cells.
   3. Tumor cells can evade immune surveillance by downregulating expression of MHC class I.
   4. Immunodeficiency (both primary and secondary) increases risk for cancer.

TUMOR PROGRESSION

I. **TUMOR INVASION AND SPREAD**
   A. Accumulation of mutations eventually results in tumor invasion and spread.
      1. Epithelial tumor cells are normally attached to one another by cellular adhesion molecules (e.g., E-cadherin).
      2. Downregulation of E-cadherin leads to dissociation of attached cells.
      3. Cells attach to laminin and destroy basement membrane (collagen type IV) via collagenase.
      4. Cells attach to fibronectin in the extracellular matrix and spread locally.
      5. Entrance into vascular or lymphatic spaces allows for metastasis (distant spread).

II. **ROUTES OF METASTASIS**
   A. Lymphatic spread is characteristic of carcinomas.
      1. Initial spread is to regional draining lymph nodes (Fig. 3.2).
   B. Hematogenous spread is characteristic of sarcomas and some carcinomas.
      1. Renal cell carcinoma (often invades renal vein)
      2. Hepatocellular carcinoma (often invades hepatic vein)
      3. Follicular carcinoma of the thyroid
      4. Choriocarcinoma
   C. Seeding of body cavities is characteristic of ovarian carcinoma, which often involves the peritoneum ('omental caking', Fig. 3.3).

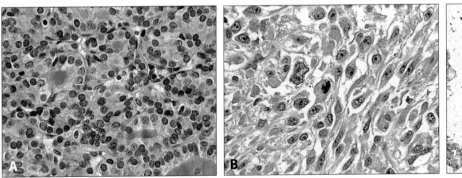

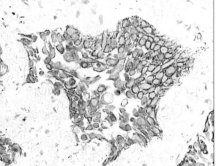

Fig. 3.4 Histologic features of neoplasia. **A,** Well differentiated, follicular adenoma of thyroid. **B,** Poorly differentiated, anaplastic carcinoma of thyroid.

Fig. 3.5 Immunohistochemical stain for keratin marking epithelial cells (in brown).

CLINICAL CHARACTERISTICS

I. **CLINICAL FEATURES**

    A. Benign tumors tend to be slow growing, well circumscribed, distinct, and mobile.

    B. Malignant tumors are usually rapid growing, poorly circumscribed, infiltrative, and fixed to surrounding tissues and local structures.

    C. Biopsy or excision is generally required before a tumor can be classified as benign or malignant with certainty.

        1. Some benign tumors can grow in a malignant-like fashion, and some malignant tumors can grow in a benign-like fashion.

II. **HISTOLOGIC FEATURES**

    A. Benign tumors are usually well differentiated (Fig. 3.4A). Characteristics include

        1. Organized growth

        2. Uniform nuclei

        3. Low nuclear to cytoplasmic ratio

        4. Minimal mitotic activity

        5. Lack of invasion (of basement membrane or local tissue)

        6. No metastatic potential

    B. Malignant tumors are classically poorly differentiated (anaplastic, Fig. 3.4B). Characteristics include

        1. Disorganized growth (loss of polarity)

        2. Nuclear pleomorphism and hyperchromasia

        3. High nuclear to cytoplasmic ratio

        4. High mitotic activity with atypical mitosis

        5. Invasion (through basement membrane or into local tissue)

    C. Metastatic potential is the hallmark of malignancy—benign tumors never metastasize.

Table 3.4: Common Immunohistochemical Stains and Target Cell Types

IMMUNOHISTOCHEMICAL STAIN	TISSUE TYPE
INTERMEDIATE FILAMENTS	
Keratin	Epithelium
Vimentin	Mesenchyme
Desmin	Muscle
GFAP	Neuroglia
Neurofilament	Neurons
OTHERS	
PSA	Prostatic epithelium
ER	Breast epithelium
Thyroglobulin	Thyroid follicular cells
Chromogranin	Neuroendocrine cells (e.g., small cell carcinoma of lung and carcinoid tumors)
S-100	Melanoma, Schwannoma and Langerhans cell histiocytosis

D. Immunohistochemistry is used to characterize tumors that are difficult to classify on histology (Fig. 3.5, Table 3.4).

III. SERUM TUMOR MARKERS

A. Proteins released by tumor into serum (e.g., PSA)

B. Useful for screening, monitoring response to treatment, and monitoring recurrence

C. Elevated levels require tissue biopsy for diagnosis of carcinoma (e.g., biopsy of prostate with elevated PSA).

IV. GRADING OF CANCER

A. Microscopic assessment of differentiation (i.e., how much a cancer resembles the tissue in which it grows); takes into account architectural and nuclear features

1. Well differentiated (low grade)—resembles normal parent tissue
2. Poorly differentiated (high grade)—does not resemble parent tissue

B. Important for determining prognosis; well-differentiated cancers have better prognosis than poorly-differentiated cancers.

V. STAGING OF CANCER

A. Assessment of size and spread of a cancer

B. Key prognostic factor; more important than grade

C. Determined after final surgical resection of the tumor

D. Utilizes TNM staging system

1. T—tumor (size and/or depth of invasion)
2. N—spread to regional lymph nodes; second most important prognostic factor
3. M—metastasis; single most important prognostic factor

Hemostasis and Related Disorders

4

INTRODUCTION

I. **HEMOSTASIS**
   A. Integrity of the blood vessel is necessary to carry blood to tissues.
      1. Damage to the wall is repaired by hemostasis, which involves formation of a thrombus (clot) at the site of vessel injury.
   B. Hemostasis occurs in two stages: primary and secondary.
      1. Primary hemostasis forms a weak platelet plug and is mediated by interaction between platelets and the vessel wall.
      2. Secondary hemostasis stabilizes the platelet plug and is mediated by the coagulation cascade.

PRIMARY HEMOSTASIS AND RELATED BLEEDING DISORDERS

I. **PRIMARY HEMOSTASIS**
   A. Step 1—Transient vasoconstriction of damaged vessel
      1. Mediated by reflex neural stimulation and endothelin release from endothelial cells
   B. Step 2—Platelet adhesion to the surface of disrupted vessel
      1. Von Willebrand factor (vWF) binds exposed subendothelial collagen.
      2. Platelets bind vWF using the GPIb receptor.
      3. vWF is derived from the Weibel-Palade bodies of endothelial cells and α-granules of platelets.
   C. Step 3—Platelet degranulation
      1. Adhesion induces shape change in platelets and degranulation with release of multiple mediators.
         i. ADP is released from platelet dense granules; promotes exposure of GPIIb/IIIa receptor on platelets.
         ii. TXA_2 is synthesized by platelet cyclooxygenase (COX) and released; promotes platelet aggregation
   D. Step 4—Platelet aggregation
      1. Platelets aggregate at the site of injury via GPIIb/IIIa using fibrinogen (from plasma) as a linking molecule; results in formation of platelet plug
      2. Platelet plug is weak; coagulation cascade (secondary hemostasis) stabilizes it.

II. **DISORDERS OF PRIMARY HEMOSTASIS**
   A. Usually due to abnormalities in platelets; divided into quantitative or qualitative disorders
   B. Clinical features include mucosal and skin bleeding.
      1. Symptoms of mucosal bleeding include epistaxis (most common overall symptom), hemoptysis, GI bleeding, hematuria, and menorrhagia. Intracranial bleeding occurs with severe thrombocytopenia.
      2. Symptoms of skin bleeding include petechiae (1–2 mm, Fig. 4.1), purpura (> 3 mm), ecchymoses (> 1 cm), and easy bruising; petechiae are a sign of thrombocytopenia and are not usually seen with qualitative disorders.

C. Useful laboratory studies include
1. Platelet count—normal 150–400 K/µL; < 50 K/µL leads to symptoms.
2. Bleeding time—normal 2–7 minutes; prolonged with quantitative and qualitative platelet disorders
3. Blood smear—used to assess number and size of platelets
4. Bone marrow biopsy—used to assess megakaryocytes, which produce platelets

III. IMMUNE THROMBOCYTOPENIC PURPURA (ITP)

A. Autoimmune production of IgG against platelet antigens (e.g., GPIIb/IIIa)
1. Most common cause of thrombocytopenia in children and adults
B. Autoantibodies are produced by plasma cells in the spleen.
C. Antibody-bound platelets are consumed by splenic macrophages, resulting in thrombocytopenia.
D. Divided into acute and chronic forms
1. Acute form arises in children weeks after a viral infection or immunization; self-limited, usually resolving within weeks of presentation
2. Chronic form arises in adults, usually women of childbearing age. May be primary or secondary (e.g., SLE). May cause short-lived thrombocytopenia in offspring since antiplatelet IgG can cross the placenta.
E. Laboratory findings include
1. ↓ platelet count, often < 50 K/µL
2. Normal PT/PTT—Coagulation factors are not affected.
3. ↑ megakaryocytes on bone marrow biopsy
F. Initial treatment is corticosteroids. Children respond well; adults may show early response, but often relapse.
1. IVIG is used to raise the platelet count in symptomatic bleeding, but its effect is short-lived.

IV
Immunoglobulin

2. Splenectomy eliminates the primary source of antibody and the site of platelet destruction (performed in refractory cases).

IV. MICROANGIOPATHIC HEMOLYTIC ANEMIA

A. Pathologic formation of platelet microthrombi in small vessels
1. Platelets are consumed in the formation of microthrombi.
2. RBCs are "sheared" as they cross microthrombi, resulting in hemolytic anemia with schistocytes (Fig. 4.2).
B. Seen in thrombotic thrombocytopenic purpura (TTP) and hemolytic uremic syndrome (HUS)
C. TTP is due to decreased ADAMTS13, an enzyme that normally cleaves vWF multimers into smaller monomers for eventual degradation.

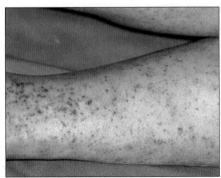

Fig. 4.1 Petechiae involving skin.

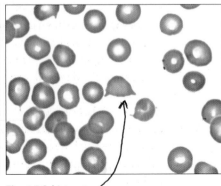

Fig. 4.2 Schistocyte.

1. Large, uncleaved multimers lead to abnormal platelet adhesion, resulting in microthrombi.
2. Decreased ADAMTS13 is usually due to an acquired autoantibody; most commonly seen in adult females

D. HUS is due to endothelial damage by drugs or infection.
  1. Classically seen in children with *E coli* O157:H7 dysentery, which results from exposure to undercooked beef
  2. *E coli* verotoxin damages endothelial cells resulting in platelet microthrombi.

E. Clinical findings (HUS and TTP) include
  1. Skin and mucosal bleeding *b/c you are thrombocytopenia*
  2. Microangiopathic hemolytic anemia
  3. Fever
  4. Renal insufficiency (more common in HUS)—Thrombi involve vessels of the kidney.
  both disorders 5. CNS abnormalities (more common in TTP)—Thrombi involve vessels of the CNS.

F. Laboratory findings include
  1. Thrombocytopenia with $\uparrow$ bleeding time
  2. Normal PT/PTT (coagulation cascade is not activated)
  3. Anemia with schistocytes
  4. $\uparrow$ megakaryocytes on bone marrow biopsy

G. Treatment involves plasmapheresis and corticosteroids, particularly in TTP.
  (used to remove protein/Ab from blood)

V. **QUALITATIVE PLATELET DISORDERS**
  A. Bernard-Soulier syndrome is due to a genetic GPIb deficiency; platelet adhesion is impaired.
    1. Blood smear shows mild thrombocytopenia with enlarged platelets. *(Big Suckers)*
  B. Glanzmann thrombasthenia is due to a genetic GPIIb/IIIa deficiency; platelet aggregation is impaired.
  C. Aspirin irreversibly inactivates cyclooxygenase; lack of TXA_2 impairs aggregation.
  D. Uremia disrupts platelet function; both adhesion and aggregation are impaired.
    $\rightarrow \uparrow$ Nitrogenous waste products   *TXA_2 brings in other platelets*

SECONDARY HEMOSTASIS AND RELATED DISORDERS

I. **SECONDARY HEMOSTASIS**
  A. Stabilizes the weak platelet plug via the coagulation cascade
    1. Coagulation cascade generates thrombin, which converts fibrinogen in the platelet plug to fibrin.
    2. Fibrin is then cross-linked, yielding a stable platelet-fibrin thrombus.
  B. Factors of the coagulation cascade are produced by the liver in an inactive state. Activation requires
    1. Exposure to an activating substance
      i. Tissue thromboplastin activates factor VII (extrinsic pathway).
      ii. Subendothelial collagen activates factor XII (intrinsic pathway).
    2. Phospholipid surface of platelets
    3. Calcium (derived from platelet dense granules)

II. **DISORDERS OF SECONDARY HEMOSTASIS**
  A. Usually due to factor abnormalities
  B. Clinical features include deep tissue bleeding into muscles and joints (hemarthrosis) and rebleeding after surgical procedures (e.g., circumcision and wisdom tooth extraction).
  C. Laboratory studies include

1. Prothrombin time (PT)—measures extrinsic (factor VII) and common (factors II, V, X, and fibrinogen) pathways of the coagulation cascade
2. Partial thromboplastin time (PTT)—measures intrinsic (factors XII, XI, IX, VIII) and common (factors II, V, X, and fibrinogen) pathways of the coagulation cascade

for (Hep) heparin

III. HEMOPHILIA A

A. Genetic factor VIII (FVIII) deficiency
   1. X-linked recessive (predominantly affects males)
   2. Can arise from a new mutation (de novo) without any family history
B. Presents with deep tissue, joint, and postsurgical bleeding
   1. Clinical severity depends on the degree of deficiency.
C. Laboratory findings include
   1. ↑PTT; normal PT
   2. ↓FVIII
   3. Normal platelet count and bleeding time
D. Treatment involves recombinant FVIII.

IV. HEMOPHILIA B (CHRISTMAS DISEASE)

A. Genetic factor IX deficiency
   1. Resembles hemophilia A, except FIX levels are decreased instead of FVIII

V. COAGULATION FACTOR INHIBITOR

A. Acquired antibody against a coagulation factor resulting in impaired factor function; anti-FVIII is most common.
   1. Clinical and lab findings are similar to hemophilia A.
   2. PTT does not correct upon mixing normal plasma with patient's plasma (mixing study) due to inhibitor; PTT does correct in hemophilia A.

VI. VON WILLEBRAND DISEASE

A. Genetic vWF deficiency
   1. Most common inherited coagulation disorder
B. Multiple subtypes exist, causing quantitative and qualitative defects; the most common type is autosomal dominant with decreased vWF levels.
C. Presents with mild mucosal and skin bleeding; low vWF impairs platelet adhesion.
D. Laboratory findings include
   1. ↑bleeding time
   2. ↑PTT; normal PT—Decreased FVIII half-life (vWF normally stabilizes FVIII); however, deep tissue, joint, and postsurgical bleeding are usually not seen. *b/c vWF stabilizes factor 8*
   3. Abnormal ristocetin test—Ristocetin induces platelet agglutination by causing vWF to bind platelet GPIb; lack of vWF → impaired agglutination → abnormal test.
E. Treatment is desmopressin (ADH analog), which increases vWF release from Weibel-Palade bodies of endothelial cells.

VII. VITAMIN K DEFICIENCY

A. Disrupts function of multiple coagulation factors *Warfarin*
   1. Vitamin K is activated by epoxide reductase in the liver.
   2. Activated vitamin K gamma carboxylates factors II, VII, IX, X, and proteins C and S; gamma carboxylation is necessary for factor function.
B. Deficiency occurs in

1. Newborns—due to lack of GI colonization by bacteria that normally synthesize vitamin K; vitamin K injection is given prophylactically to all newborns at birth to prevent hemorrhagic disease of the newborn.
2. Long-term antibiotic therapy—disrupts vitamin K-producing bacteria in the GI tract
3. Malabsorption—leads to deficiency of fat-soluble vitamins, including vitamin K

VIII. **OTHER CAUSES OF ABNORMAL SECONDARY HEMOSTASIS**
   A. Liver failure—decreased production of coagulation factors and decreased activation of vitamin K by epoxide reductase; effect of liver failure on coagulation is followed using PT.
   B. Large-volume transfusion—dilutes coagulation factors, resulting in a relative deficiency

OTHER DISORDERS OF HEMOSTASIS

I. **HEPARIN-INDUCED THROMBOCYTOPENIA**
   A. Platelet destruction that arises secondary to heparin therapy
   B. Fragments of destroyed platelets may activate remaining platelets, leading to thrombosis.   *Hep complexes w/ PF4*
      ↳ don't give warfarin

II. **DISSEMINATED INTRAVASCULAR COAGULATION** (DIC)
   A. Pathologic activation of the coagulation cascade
      1. Widespread microthrombi result in ischemia and infarction.
      2. Consumption of platelets and factors results in bleeding, especially from IV sites and mucosal surfaces (bleeding from body orifices).
   B. Almost always secondary to another disease process
      1. Obstetric complications—Tissue thromboplastin in the amniotic fluid activates coagulation.
      2. Sepsis (especially with *E Coli* or *N meningitidis*)—Endotoxins from the bacterial wall and cytokines (e.g., TNF and IL-1) induce endothelial cells to make tissue factor.
      3. Adenocarcinoma—Mucin activates coagulation.
      4. Acute promyelocytic leukemia—Primary granules activate coagulation.
      5. Rattlesnake bite—Venom activates coagulation.
   C. Laboratory findings include
      1. ↓ platelet count
      2. ↑ PT/PTT
      3. ↓ fibrinogen
      4. Microangiopathic hemolytic anemia
      5. Elevated fibrin split products, particularly D-dimer   *D-dimer = produced by lysis of crosslinked fibrin*
         i. Elevated D-dimer is the best screening test for DIC.
         ii. Derived from splitting of cross-linked fibrin; D-dimer is not produced from splitting of fibrinogen.
   D. Treatment involves addressing the underlying cause and transfusing blood products and cryoprecipitate (contains coagulation factors), as necessary.

III. **DISORDERS OF FIBRINOLYSIS**
   A. Normal fibrinolysis removes thrombus after damaged vessel heals.
      1. Tissue plasminogen activator (tPA) converts plasminogen to plasmin.
      2. Plasmin cleaves fibrin and serum fibrinogen, destroys coagulation factors, and blocks platelet aggregation.
      3. α2-antiplasmin inactivates plasmin.

B. Disorders of fibrinolysis are due to plasmin overactivity resulting in excessive cleavage of serum fibrinogen. Examples include
    1. Radical prostatectomy—Release of urokinase activates plasmin.
    2. Cirrhosis of liver—reduced production of α2-antiplasmin
C. Presents with increased bleeding (resembles DIC)
D. Laboratory findings include
    1. ↑ PT/PTT—Plasmin destroys coagulation factors.
    2. ↑ bleeding time with normal platelet count—Plasmin blocks platelet aggregation.
    3. Increased fibrinogen split products without D-dimers—Serum fibrinogen is lysed; however, D-dimers are not formed because fibrin thrombi are absent.
E. Treatment is aminocaproic acid, which blocks activation of plasminogen.

THROMBOSIS

I. **BASIC PRINCIPLES**
    A. Pathologic formation of an intravascular blood clot (thrombus)
        1. Can occur in an artery or vein
        2. Most common location is the deep veins (DVT) of the leg below the knee.
    B. Characterized by (1) lines of Zahn (alternating layers of platelets/fibrin and RBCs, Fig. 4.3) and (2) attachment to vessel wall
        1. Both features distinguish thrombus from postmortem clot.
    C. Three major risk factors for thrombosis are disruption in blood flow, endothelial cell damage, and hypercoagulable state (Virchow triad).

II. **DISRUPTION IN NORMAL BLOOD FLOW**
    A. Stasis and turbulence of blood flow increases risk for thrombosis.
        1. Blood flow is normally continuous and laminar; keeps platelets and factors dispersed and inactivated
    B. Examples include
        1. Immobilization—increased risk for deep venous thrombosis
        2. Cardiac wall dysfunction (e.g., arrhythmia or myocardial infarction)
        3. Aneurysm

III. **ENDOTHELIAL CELL DAMAGE**
    A. Endothelial damage disrupts the protective function of endothelial cells, increasing the risk for thrombosis.
    B. Endothelial cells prevent thrombosis by several mechanisms.
        1. Block exposure to subendothelial collagen and underlying tissue factor
        2. Produce prostacyclin (PGI_2) and NO—vasodilation and inhibition of platelet aggregation

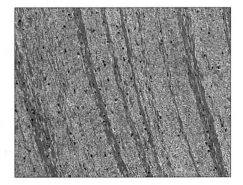

Fig. 4.3 Lines of Zahn characterized by alternating layers of platelets/fibrin and RBCs.

3. Secrete heparin-like molecules—augment antithrombin III (ATIII), which inactivates thrombin and coagulation factors
4. Secrete tissue plasminogen activator (tPA)—converts plasminogen to plasmin, which (1) cleaves fibrin and serum fibrinogen, (2) destroys coagulation factors, and (3) blocks platelet aggregation
5. Secrete thrombomodulin—redirects thrombin to activate protein C, which inactivates factors V and VIII

C. Causes of endothelial cell damage include atherosclerosis, vasculitis, and high levels of homocysteine.
   1. Vitamin B12 and folate deficiency result in mildly elevated homocysteine levels, increasing the risk for thrombosis.
      i. Folic acid (tetrahydrofolate, THF) circulates as methyl-THF in the serum.
      ii. Methyl is transferred to cobalamin (vitamin B12), allowing THF to participate in the synthesis of DNA precursors.
      iii. Cobalamin transfers methyl to homocysteine resulting in methionine.
      iv. Lack of vitamin B12 or folate leads to decreased conversion of homocysteine to methionine resulting in buildup of homocysteine.
   2. Cystathionine beta synthase (CBS) deficiency results in high homocysteine levels with homocystinuria.
      i. CBS converts homocysteine to cystathionine; enzyme deficiency leads to homocysteine buildup.
      ii. Characterized by vessel thrombosis, mental retardation, lens dislocation, and long slender fingers.

IV. HYPERCOAGULABLE STATE

A. Due to excessive procoagulant proteins or defective anticoagulant proteins; may be inherited or acquired
B. Classic presentation is recurrent DVTs or DVT at a young age.
   1. Usually occurs in the deep veins of the leg; other sites include hepatic and cerebral veins.
C. Protein C or S deficiency (autosomal dominant) decreases negative feedback on the coagulation cascade.
   1. Proteins C and S normally inactivate factors V and VIII.
   2. Increased risk for warfarin skin necrosis
      i. Initial stage of warfarin therapy results in a temporary deficiency of proteins C and S (due to shorter half-life) relative to factors II, VII, IX, and X
      ii. In preexisting C or S deficiency, a severe deficiency is seen at the onset of warfarin therapy increasing risk for thrombosis, especially in the skin.
D. Factor V Leiden is a mutated form of factor V that lacks the cleavage site for deactivation by proteins C and S.
   1. Most common inherited cause of hypercoagulable state
E. Prothrombin 20210A is an inherited point mutation in prothrombin that results in increased gene expression.
   1. Increased prothrombin results in increased thrombin, promoting thrombus formation.
F. ATIII deficiency decreases the protective effect of heparin-like molecules produced by the endothelium, increasing the risk for thrombus.
   1. Heparin-like molecules normally activate ATIII, which inactivates thrombin and coagulation factors.
   2. In ATIII deficiency, PTT does not rise with standard heparin dosing.
      i. Pharmacologic heparin works by binding and activating ATIII.
      ii. High doses of heparin activate limited ATIII; coumadin is then given to maintain an anticoagulated state.

G. Oral contraceptives are associated with a hypercoagulable state.
   1. Estrogen induces increased production of coagulation factors, thereby increasing the risk for thrombosis.

EMBOLISM

I. **BASIC PRINCIPLES**
   A. Intravascular mass that travels and occludes downstream vessels; symptoms depend on the vessel involved.
   B. Thromboembolus is due to a thrombus that dislodges; most common type of embolus (>95%)
   C. Atherosclerotic embolus is due to an atherosclerotic plaque that dislodges.
      1. Characterized by the presence of cholesterol clefts in the embolus (Fig. 4.4A)
   D. Fat embolus is associated with bone fractures, particularly long bones, and soft tissue trauma.
      1. Develops while fracture is still present or shortly after repair
      2. Characterized by dyspnea (fat, often with bone marrow elements, is seen in pulmonary vessels, Fig. 4.4B) and petechiae on the skin overlying the chest
   E. Gas embolus is classically seen in decompression sickness.
      1. Nitrogen gas precipitates out of blood due to rapid ascent by a diver.
      2. Presents with joint and muscle pain ('bends') and respiratory symptoms ('chokes').
      3. Chronic form (Caisson disease) is characterized by multifocal ischemic necrosis of bone.
      4. Gas embolus may also occur during laparoscopic surgery (air is pumped into the abdomen).
   F. Amniotic fluid embolus enters maternal circulation during labor or delivery
      1. Presents with shortness of breath, neurologic symptoms, and DIC (due to the thrombogenic nature of amniotic fluid)
      2. Characterized by squamous cells and keratin debris, from fetal skin, in embolus (Fig. 4.4C)

II. **PULMONARY EMBOLISM (PE)**
   A. Usually due to thromboembolus; the most common source is deep venous thrombus (DVT) of the lower extremity, usually involving the femoral, iliac, or popliteal veins.
   B. Most often clinically silent because (1) the lung has a dual blood supply (via pulmonary and bronchial arteries) and (2) the embolus is usually small (self-resolves)

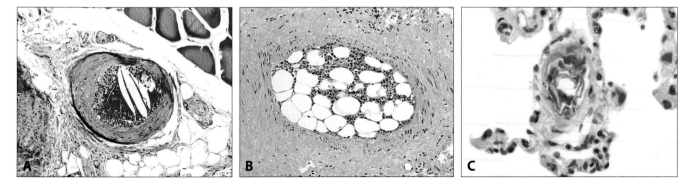

Fig. 4.4 Emboli. **A**, Atherosclerotic embolus characterized by cholesterol clefts. **B**, Fat embolus with bone marrow elements. **C**, Amniotic fluid embolus with squamous cells and keratin debris from fetal skin. (A, Courtesy of Professor A. Garfia. C, Courtesy of Shakuntala Teas, MD)

C. Pulmonary infarction occurs if a large- or medium-sized artery is obstructed in patients with pre-existing cardiopulmonary compromise; only 10% of PEs cause infarction.
　1. Presents with shortness of breath, hemoptysis, pleuritic chest pain, and pleural effusion
　2. V/Q lung scan shows mismatch; perfusion is abnormal.
　3. Spiral CT shows a vascular filling defect in the lung.
　4. Lower extremity Doppler ultrasound is useful to detect DVT.
　5. D-dimer is elevated.
　6. Gross examination reveals a hemorrhagic, wedge-shaped infarct.
D. Sudden death occurs with a large saddle embolus that blocks both left and right pulmonary arteries or with significant occlusion of a large pulmonary artery (Fig. 4.5); death is due to electromechanical dissociation.
E. Pulmonary hypertension may arise with chronic emboli that are reorganized over time.

III. **SYSTEMIC EMBOLISM**
A. Usually due to thromboembolus
B. Most commonly arise in the left heart
C. Travel down systemic circulation to occlude flow to organs, most commonly the lower extremities

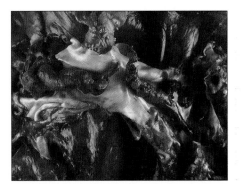

Fig. 4.5 Saddle embolus involving pulmonary artery. (Courtesy of Yale Rosen, MD)

Red Blood Cell Disorders

5

ANEMIA

I. **BASIC PRINCIPLES**
   A. Reduction in circulating red blood cell (RBC) mass
   B. Presents with signs and symptoms of hypoxia
      1. Weakness, fatigue, and dyspnea
      2. Pale conjunctiva and skin
      3. Headache and lightheadedness
      4. Angina, especially with preexisting coronary artery disease
   C. Hemoglobin (Hb), hematocrit (Hct), and RBC count are used as surrogates for RBC mass, which is difficult to measure.
      1. Anemia is defined as Hb < 13.5 g/dL in males and < 12.5 g/dL in females (normal Hb is 13.5–17.5 g/dL in males and 12.5–16.0 g/dL in females).
   D. Based on mean corpuscular volume (MCV), anemia can be classified as microcytic (MCV < 80 μm^3), normocytic (MCV = 80–100 μm^3), or macrocytic (MCV > 100 μm^3).

← > normal   *MCV = size of RBC*

MICROCYTIC ANEMIAS = *low Hb*

erythroblast is large + divides multiple times to create small RBC's

I. **BASIC PRINCIPLES**
   A. Anemia with MCV < 80 μm^3
   B. Microcytic anemias are due to decreased production of hemoglobin.
      1. RBC progenitor cells in the bone marrow are large and normally divide multiple times to produce smaller mature cells (MCV = 80–100 μm^3).
      2. Microcytosis is due to an "extra" division which occurs to maintain hemoglobin concentration.
   C. Hemoglobin is made of heme and globin; heme is composed of iron and protoporphyrin. A decrease in any of these components leads to microcytic anemia.
   D. Microcytic anemias include (1) iron deficiency anemia, (2) anemia of chronic disease, (3) sideroblastic anemia, and (4) thalassemia.

II. **IRON DEFICIENCY ANEMIA**
   A. Due to decreased levels of iron
      1. ↓ iron → ↓ heme → ↓ hemoglobin → microcytic anemia
   B. Most common type of anemia
      1. Lack of iron is the most common nutritional deficiency in the world, affecting roughly 1/3 of world's population.
   C. Iron is consumed in heme (meat-derived) and non-heme (vegetable-derived) forms.
      1. Absorption occurs in the duodenum. Enterocytes have heme and non-heme (DMT1) transporters; the heme form is more readily absorbed.
      2. Enterocytes transport iron across the cell membrane into blood via ferroportin.
      3. Transferrin transports iron in the blood and delivers it to liver and bone marrow macrophages for storage.
      4. Stored intracellular iron is bound to ferritin, which prevents iron from forming free radicals via the Fenton reaction.

body can't really excrete Fe

D. Laboratory measurements of iron status
1. Serum iron—measure of iron in the blood
2. Total iron-binding capacity (TIBC)—measure of transferrin molecules in the blood
3. % saturation—percentage of transferrin molecules that are bound by iron (normal is 33%)
4. Serum ferritin—reflects iron stores in macrophages and the liver

E. Iron deficiency is usually caused by dietary lack or blood loss.
1. Infants—breast-feeding (human milk is low in iron)
2. Children—poor diet
3. Adults (20–50 years)—peptic ulcer disease in males and menorrhagia or pregnancy in females
4. Elderly—colon polyps/carcinoma in the Western world; hookworm (*Ancylostoma duodenale* and *Necator americanus*) in the developing world
5. Other causes include malnutrition, malabsorption, and gastrectomy (acid aids iron absorption by maintaining the Fe^{2+} state, which is more readily absorbed than Fe^{3+}).

Fe² goes in2 the body
↗ opposite always

F. Stages of iron deficiency
1. Storage iron is depleted—↓ ferritin; ↑ TIBC
2. Serum iron is depleted—↓ serum iron; ↓ % saturation
3. Normocytic anemia—Bone marrow makes fewer, but normal-sized, RBCs.
4. Microcytic, hypochromic anemia—Bone marrow makes smaller and fewer RBCs.

G. Clinical features of iron deficiency include anemia, koilonychia, and pica. *→ eat dirt or ice*

H. Laboratory findings include
1. Microcytic, hypochromic RBCs with ↑ red cell distribution width (RDW, Fig. 5.1)
   ↳ spread of RBC size
2. ↓ ferritin; ↑ TIBC; ↓ serum iron; ↓ % saturation
3. ↑ Free erythrocyte protoporphyrin (FEP)

I. Treatment involves supplemental iron (ferrous sulfate).
J. Plummer-Vinson syndrome is iron deficiency anemia with esophageal web and atrophic glossitis; presents as anemia, dysphagia, and beefy-red tongue

hypochromic = ↓ color

normal RBCs should be ≈ the size of leukocyte nucleus

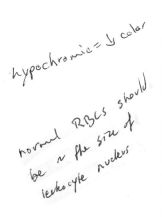

III. ANEMIA OF CHRONIC DISEASE

A. Anemia associated with chronic inflammation (e.g., endocarditis or autoimmune conditions) or cancer; most common type of anemia in hospitalized patients
B. Chronic disease results in production of acute phase reactants from the liver, including hepcidin.
1. Hepcidin sequesters iron in storage sites by (1) limiting iron transfer from macrophages to erythroid precursors and (2) suppressing erythropoietin (EPO)

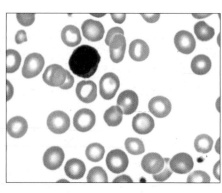

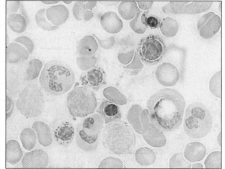

Fig. 5.1 Microcytic, hypochromic RBCs of iron deficiency anemia.

Fig. 5.2 Ringed sideroblasts (Prussian blue stain).

production; aim is to prevent bacteria from accessing iron, which is necessary for their survival.

   2. ↓ available iron → ↓ heme → ↓ hemoglobin → microcytic anemia

  C. Laboratory findings include *↓normocytic anemia↗*

   1. ↑ ferritin, ↓ TIBC, ↓ serum iron, and ↓ % saturation

   2. ↑ Free erythrocyte protoporphyrin (FEP)

  D. Treatment involves addressing the underlying cause.

IV. SIDEROBLASTIC ANEMIA

  A. Anemia due to defective protoporphyrin synthesis

   1. ↓ protoporphyrin → ↓ heme → ↓ hemoglobin → microcytic anemia

  B. Protoporphyrin is synthesized via a series of reactions.

   1. Aminolevulinic acid synthetase (ALAS) converts succinyl CoA to aminolevulinic acid (ALA) using vitamin B6 as a cofactor (rate-limiting step).

   2. Aminolevulinic acid dehydratase (ALAD) converts ALA to porphobilinogen.

   3. Additional reactions convert porphobilinogen to protoporphyrin.

   4. Ferrochelatase attaches protoporphyrin to iron to make heme (final reaction; occurs in the mitochondria).

  C. Iron is transferred to erythroid precursors and enters the mitochondria to form heme. If protoporphyrin is deficient, iron remains trapped in mitochondria.

   1. Iron-laden mitochondria form a ring around the nucleus of erythroid precursors; these cells are called ringed sideroblasts (hence, the term sideroblastic anemia, Fig. 5.2). *↳ in bone marrow biopsy*

  D. Sideroblastic anemia can be congenital or acquired.

   1. Congenital defect most commonly involves ALAS (rate-limiting enzyme).

   2. Acquired causes include

    i. Alcoholism—mitochondrial poison

    ii. Lead poisoning—inhibits ALAD and ferrochelatase

    iii. Vitamin B6 deficiency—required cofactor for ALAS; most commonly seen as a side effect of isoniazid treatment for tuberculosis

  E. Laboratory findings include ↑ ferritin, ↓ TIBC, ↑ serum iron, and ↑ % saturation (iron-overloaded state). *↳ like hemochromatosis*

V. THALASSEMIA

  A. Anemia due to decreased synthesis of the globin chains of hemoglobin

   1. ↓ globin → ↓ hemoglobin → microcytic anemia

  B. Inherited mutation; carriers are protected against *Plasmodium falciparum* malaria.

  C. Divided into α- and β-thalassemia based on decreased production of alpha or beta globin chains.

   1. Normal types of hemoglobin are HbF ($\alpha_2\gamma_2$) *fetal*, HbA ($\alpha_2\beta_2$), and HbA$_2$ ($\alpha_2\delta_2$) *delta*.

α is most important

Handwritten margin notes:
Succinyl CoA
↓ ALAS + B₆
ALA
↓ ALAD
porphobilinogen
↓
↓
Porphobilinogen
↓
protoporphyrin → mitochondria
Ferrochelatase ↗
protoporphyrin + Fe = heme

Prussian blue stain = Fe

Lead denatures proteins

Table 5.1: Laboratory Findings in Microcytic Anemia

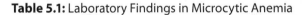

STATE	FERRITIN	TIBC	SERUM IRON	% SATURATION
Normal	–	300 µg/dL	100 µg/dL	33%
Iron Deficiency Anemia	Low	High	Low	Low
Anemia of Chronic Disease	High	Low	Low	Low
Sideroblastic Anemia	High	Low	High	High
Pregnancy and oral contraceptives	–	High	–	Low

D. α-Thalassemia is usually due to gene deletion; normally, 4 alpha genes are present on chromosome 16. (2 on each chromosome)

1. One gene deleted—asymptomatic

2. Two genes deleted—mild anemia with ↑ RBC count; cis deletion is associated with an increased risk of severe thalassemia in offspring.

   i. Cis deletion is when both deletions occur on the same chromosome; seen in Asians (more severe)

   ii. Trans deletion is when one deletion occurs on each chromosome; seen in Africans, including African Americans

3. Three genes deleted—severe anemia; β chains form tetramers (HbH) that damage RBCs; HbH is seen on electrophoresis. ⌐$\beta_2\beta_2$

4. Four genes deleted—lethal in utero (hydrops fetalis); γ chains form tetramers (Hb Barts) that damage RBCs; Hb Barts is seen on electrophoresis.

E. β-Thalassemia is usually due to gene mutations (point mutations in promoter or splicing sites); seen in individuals of African and Mediterranean descent

1. Two β genes are present on chromosome 11; mutations result in absent (β^0) or diminished (β^+) production of the β-globin chain.

2. β-Thalassemia minor (β/β^+) is the mildest form of disease and is usually asymptomatic with an increased RBC count.

   i. Microcytic, hypochromic RBCs and target cells are seen on blood smear (Fig. 5.3).

   ii. Hemoglobin electrophoresis shows slightly decreased HbA with increased HbA$_2$ (5%, normal 2.5%) and HbF (2%, normal 1%).

3. β-Thalassemia major (β^0/β^0) is the most severe form of disease and presents with severe anemia a few months after birth; high HbF ($\alpha_2\gamma_2$) at birth is temporarily protective.

   i. α tetramers aggregate and damage RBCs, resulting in ineffective erythropoiesis and extravascular hemolysis (removal of circulating RBCs by the spleen).

   ii. Massive erythroid hyperplasia ensues resulting in (1) expansion of hematopoiesis into the skull (reactive bone formation leads to 'crewcut' appearance on x-ray, Fig. 5.4) and facial bones ('chipmunk facies'), (2) extramedullary hematopoiesis with hepatosplenomegaly, and (3) risk of aplastic crisis with parvovirus B19 infection of erythroid precursors.

   iii. Chronic transfusions are often necessary; leads to risk for secondary hemochromatosis

   iv. Smear shows microcytic, hypochromic RBCs with target cells and nucleated red blood cells.

   v. Electrophoresis shows HbA$_2$ and HbF with little or no HbA.

[handwritten margin note: Target cell ↓Hb in RBC cytosol]

[handwritten margin note: in liver to spleen]

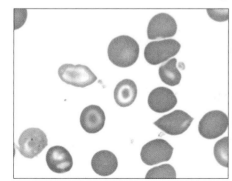

Fig. 5.3 Target cells.

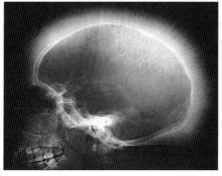

Fig. 5.4 'Crewcut' appearance. (Reproduced with permission, www.orthopaedia.com/x/xgGvAQ)

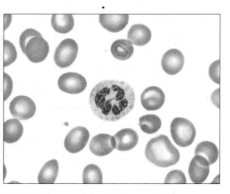

Fig. 5.5 Hypersegmented neutrophil in macrocytic anemia.

MACROCYTIC ANEMIA

I. **BASIC PRINCIPLES**
   A. Anemia with MCV > 100 μm^3; most commonly due to folate or vitamin B12 deficiency (megaloblastic anemia)
   B. Folate and vitamin B12 are necessary for synthesis of DNA precursors.
      1. Folate circulates in the serum as methyltetrahydrofolate (methyl THF); removal of the methyl group allows for participation in the synthesis of DNA precursors.
      2. Methyl group is transferred to vitamin B12 (cobalamin).
      3. Vitamin B12 then transfers it to homocysteine, producing methionine.
   C. Lack of folate or vitamin B12 impairs synthesis of DNA precursors.
      1. Impaired division and enlargement of RBC precursors leads to megaloblastic anemia.
      2. Impaired division of granulocytic precursors leads to hypersegmented neutrophils. >5 lobes
      3. Megaloblastic change is also seen in rapidly-dividing (e.g., intestinal) epithelial cells.
   D. Other causes of macrocytic anemia (without megaloblastic change) include alcoholism, liver disease, and drugs (e.g., 5-FU). ⤷ no hypersegmented PMN's

II. **FOLATE DEFICIENCY**
   A. Dietary folate is obtained from green vegetables and some fruits.
      1. Absorbed in the jejunum
   B. Folate deficiency develops within months, as body stores are minimal.
   C. Causes include poor diet (e.g., alcoholics and elderly), increased demand (e.g., pregnancy, cancer, and hemolytic anemia), and folate antagonists (e.g., methotrexate, which inhibits dihydrofolate reductase).
   D. Clinical and laboratory findings include
      1. Macrocytic RBCs and hypersegmented neutrophils (> 5 lobes, Fig. 5.5)
      2. Glossitis – inflammation of the tongue
      3. ↓ serum folate
      4. ↑ serum homocysteine (increases risk for thrombosis)
      5. Normal methylmalonic acid ⟶ Succinyl CoA
         B12

III. **VITAMIN B12 DEFICIENCY**
   A. Dietary vitamin B12 is complexed to animal-derived proteins.
      1. Salivary gland enzymes (e.g., amylase) liberate vitamin B12, which is then bound by R-binder (also from the salivary gland) and carried through the stomach.
      2. Pancreatic proteases in the duodenum detach vitamin B12 from R-binder.
      3. Vitamin B12 binds intrinsic factor (made by gastric parietal cells) in the small bowel; the intrinsic factor-vitamin B12 complex is absorbed in the ileum.
   B. Vitamin B12 deficiency is less common than folate deficiency and takes years to develop due to large hepatic stores of vitamin B12.
   C. Pernicious anemia is the most common cause of vitamin B12 deficiency.
      1. Autoimmune destruction of parietal cells (body of stomach) leads to intrinsic factor deficiency
   D. Other causes of vitamin B12 deficiency include pancreatic insufficiency and damage to the terminal ileum (e.g., Crohn disease or *Diphyllobothrium latum* [fish tapeworm]); dietary deficiency is rare, except in vegans.
   E. Clinical and laboratory findings include
      1. Macrocytic RBCs with hypersegmented neutrophils
      2. Glossitis
      3. Subacute combined degeneration of the spinal cord

     i. Vitamin B12 is a cofactor for the conversion of methylmalonic acid to succinyl CoA (important in fatty acid metabolism).

     ii. Vitamin B12 deficiency results in increased levels of methylmalonic acid, which impairs spinal cord myelinization.

     iii. Damage results in poor proprioception and vibratory sensation (posterior column) and spastic paresis (lateral corticospinal tract).

   4. ↓ serum vitamin B12

   5. ↑ serum homocysteine (similar to folate deficiency), which increases risk for thrombosis

   6. ↑ methylmalonic acid (unlike folate deficiency)

[Handwritten margin note: B12 is involved in 2 rxns ① meth transfer from THF to Homocysteine ② conversion of methylmalonic acid to succinyl CoA]

NORMOCYTIC ANEMIA

I. **BASIC PRINCIPLES**

   A. Anemia with normal-sized RBCs (MCV = 80–100 μm^3)

   B. Due to increased peripheral destruction or underproduction

     1. Reticulocyte count helps to distinguish between these two etiologies. *[handwritten: ↳ stage w/ blood]*

II. **RETICULOCYTES**

   A. Young RBCs released from the bone marrow

     1. Identified on blood smear as larger cells with bluish cytoplasm (due to residual RNA, Fig. 5.6)

   B. Normal reticulocyte count (RC) is 1–2%.

     1. RBC lifespan is 120 days; each day roughly 1–2% of RBCs are removed from circulation and replaced by reticulocytes.

   C. A properly functioning marrow responds to anemia by increasing the RC to > 3%.

   D. RC, however, is falsely elevated in anemia.

     1. RC is measured as percentage of total RBCs; decrease in total RBCs falsely elevates percentage of reticulocytes.

   E. RC is corrected by multiplying reticulocyte count by Hct/45.

     1. Corrected count > 3% indicates good marrow response and suggests peripheral destruction.

     2. Corrected count < 3% indicates poor marrow response and suggests underproduction.

III. **PERIPHERAL RBC DESTRUCTION (HEMOLYSIS)**

   A. Divided into extravascular and intravascular hemolysis; both result in anemia with a good marrow response.

   B. Extravascular hemolysis involves RBC destruction by the reticuloendothelial system (macrophages of the spleen, liver, and lymph nodes).

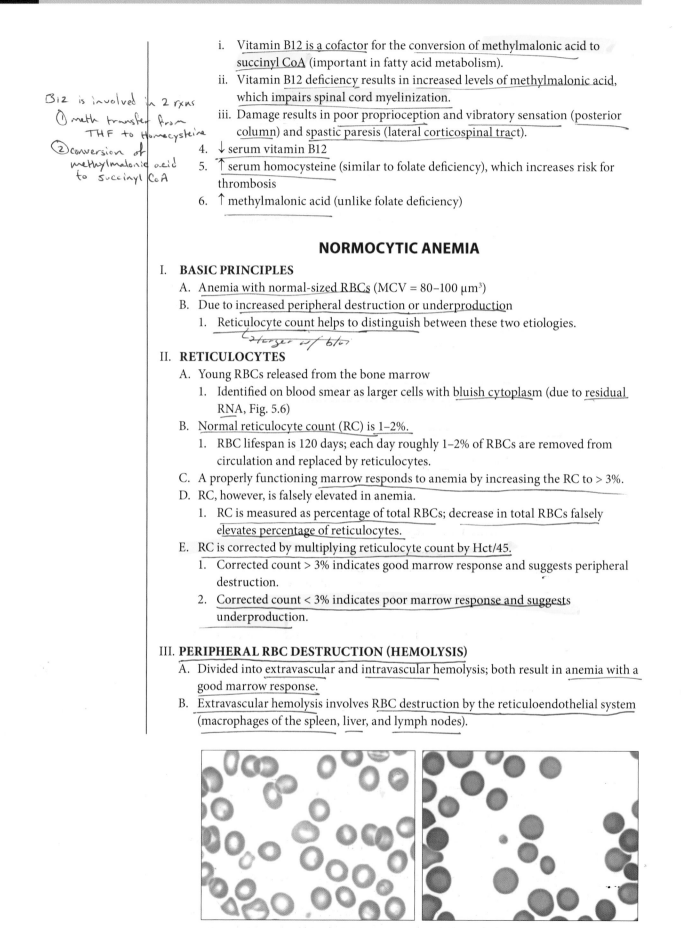

Fig. 5.6 Reticulocyte.   **Fig. 5.7** Spherocytes.

1. Macrophages consume RBCs and break down hemoglobin.
   i. Globin is broken down into amino acids.
   ii. Heme is broken down into iron and protoporphyrin; iron is recycled.
   iii. Protoporphyrin is broken down into unconjugated bilirubin, which is bound to serum albumin and delivered to the liver for conjugation and excretion into bile.
2. Clinical and laboratory findings include
   i. Anemia with splenomegaly, jaundice due to unconjugated bilirubin, and increased risk for bilirubin gallstones
   ii. Marrow hyperplasia with corrected reticulocyte count > 3%
C. Intravascular hemolysis involves destruction of RBCs within vessels.
   1. Clinical and laboratory findings include
      i. Hemoglobinemia
      ii. Hemoglobinuria
      iii. Hemosiderinuria—Renal tubular cells pick up some of the hemoglobin that is filtered into the urine and break it down into iron, which accumulates as hemosiderin; tubular cells are eventually shed resulting in hemosiderinuria.
      iv. Decreased serum haptoglobin
      └→ saves Fe in hemoglobin

NORMOCYTIC ANEMIAS WITH PREDOMINANT EXTRAVASCULAR HEMOLYSIS

I. **HEREDITARY SPHEROCYTOSIS**
   A. Inherited defect of RBC cytoskeleton-membrane tethering proteins
      1. Most commonly involves ankyrin, spectrin, or band 3
   B. Membrane blebs are formed and lost over time.
      1. Loss of membrane renders cells round (spherocytes) instead of disc-shaped.
      2. Spherocytes are less able to maneuver through splenic sinusoids and are consumed by splenic macrophages, resulting in anemia.
   C. Clinical and laboratory findings include
      1. Spherocytes with loss of central pallor (Fig. 5.7) *→ cell shrinks, but [Hb] is constant*
      2. ↑ RDW and ↑ mean corpuscular hemoglobin concentration (MCHC) *lots of variability in size*
      3. Splenomegaly, jaundice with unconjugated bilirubin, and increased risk for bilirubin gallstones (extravascular hemolysis)
      4. Increased risk for aplastic crisis with parvovirus B19 infection of erythroid precursors
   D. Diagnosed by osmotic fragility test, which reveals increased spherocyte fragility in hypotonic solution
   E. Treatment is splenectomy; anemia resolves, but spherocytes persist and Howell-Jolly bodies (fragments of nuclear material in RBCs) emerge on blood smear (Fig. 5.8).

      spleen removes nuclear small leftover fragment in RBC
      no spleen = retention of small nuclear fragments

II. **SICKLE CELL ANEMIA**
   A. Autosomal recessive mutation in β chain of hemoglobin; a single amino acid change replaces normal glutamic acid (hydrophilic) with valine (hydrophobic).
   B. Gene is carried by 10% of individuals of African descent, likely due to protective role against falciparum malaria.
   C. Sickle cell disease arises when two abnormal β genes are present; results in >90% HbS in RBCs
   D. HbS polymerizes when deoxygenated; polymers aggregate into needle-like structures, resulting in sickle cells (Fig. 5.9).
      1. Increased risk of sickling occurs with hypoxemia, dehydration, and acidosis.
      2. HbF protects against sickling; high HbF at birth is protective for the first few months of life. Treatment with hydroxyurea increases levels of HbF.

E. Cells continuously sickle and de-sickle while passing through the microcirculation, resulting in complications related to RBC membrane damage.
   1. Extravascular hemolysis—Reticuloendothelial system removes RBCs with damaged membranes, leading to anemia, jaundice with unconjugated hyperbilirubinemia, and increased risk for bilirubin gallstones.
   2. Intravascular hemolysis—RBCs with damaged membranes dehydrate, leading to hemolysis with decreased haptoglobin and target cells on blood smear.
   3. Massive erythroid hyperplasia ensues resulting in
      i. Expansion of hematopoiesis into the skull ('crewcut' appearance on x-ray) and facial bones ('chipmunk facies')
      ii. Extramedullary hematopoiesis with hepatomegaly
      iii. Risk of aplastic crisis with parvovirus B19 infection of erythroid precursors
F. Irreversible sickling leads to complications of vaso-occlusion. →infarction
   1. Dactylitis—swollen hands and feet due to vaso-occlusive infarcts in bones; common presenting sign in infants (6 months)
   2. Autosplenectomy—shrunken, fibrotic spleen. Consequences include
      i. Increased risk of infection with encapsulated organisms such as *Streptococcus pneumoniae* and *Haemophilus influenzae* (most common cause of death in children); affected children should be vaccinated by 5 years of age.
      ii. Increased risk of *Salmonella paratyphi* osteomyelitis
      iii. Howell-Jolly bodies on blood smear
   3. Acute chest syndrome—vaso-occlusion in pulmonary microcirculation
      i. Presents with chest pain, shortness of breath, and lung infiltrates
      ii. Often precipitated by pneumonia
      iii. Most common cause of death in adult patients
   4. Pain crisis
   5. Renal papillary necrosis—results in gross hematuria and proteinuria
G. Sickle cell trait is the presence of one mutated and one normal β chain; results in < 50% HbS in RBCs (HbA is slightly more efficiently produced than HbS)
   1. Generally asymptomatic with no anemia; RBCs with < 50% HbS do not sickle in vivo except in the renal medulla.
      i. Extreme hypoxia and hypertonicity of the medulla cause sickling, which results in microinfarctions leading to microscopic hematuria and, eventually, decreased ability to concentrate urine.
H. Laboratory findings
   1. Sickle cells and target cells are seen on blood smear in sickle cell disease, but not in sickle cell trait.
   2. Metabisulfite screen causes cells with any amount of HbS to sickle; positive in both disease and trait
   3. Hb electrophoresis confirms the presence and amount of HbS.

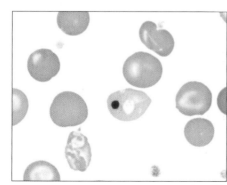

Fig. 5.8 Fragment of nuclear remnant (Howell-Jolly body) within RBC.

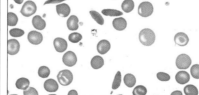

Fig. 5.9 Sickle cell disease.

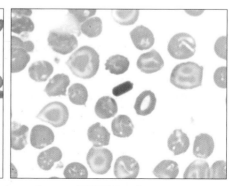

Fig. 5.10 Hemoglobin C crystal.

i. Disease—90% HbS, 8% HbF, 2% HbA$_2$ (no HbA)
ii. Trait—55% HbA, 43% HbS, 2% HbA$_2$

III. HEMOGLOBIN C
A. Autosomal recessive mutation in β chain of hemoglobin
   1. Normal glutamic acid is replaced by lysine. = C
   2. Less common than sickle cell disease
B. Presents with mild anemia due to extravascular hemolysis
C. Characteristic HbC crystals are seen in RBCs on blood smear (Fig. 5.10).

NORMOCYTIC ANEMIAS WITH PREDOMINANT INTRAVASCULAR HEMOLYSIS

I. PAROXYSMAL NOCTURNAL HEMOGLOBINURIA (PNH)
A. Acquired defect in myeloid stem cells resulting in absent glycosylphosphatidylinositol (GPI); renders cells susceptible to destruction by complement
   1. Blood cells coexist with complement.
   2. Decay accelerating factor (DAF) on the surface of blood cells protects against complement-mediated damage by inhibiting C3 convertase.
   3. DAF is secured to the cell membrane by GPI (an anchoring protein).
   4. Absence of GPI leads to absence of DAF, rendering cells susceptible to complement-mediated damage.
B. Intravascular hemolysis occurs episodically, often at night during sleep.
   1. Mild respiratory acidosis develops with shallow breathing during sleep and activates complement.
   2. RBCs, WBCs, and platelets are lysed.
   3. Intravascular hemolysis leads to hemoglobinemia and hemoglobinuria (especially in the morning); hemosiderinuria is seen days after hemolysis.
C. Sucrose test is used to screen for disease; confirmatory test is the acidified serum test or flow cytometry to detect lack of CD55 (DAF) on blood cells.
D. Main cause of death is thrombosis of the hepatic, portal, or cerebral veins.
   1. Destroyed platelets release cytoplasmic contents into circulation, inducing thrombosis.
E. Complications include iron deficiency anemia (due to chronic loss of hemoglobin in the urine) and acute myeloid leukemia (AML), which develops in 10% of patients.

II. GLUCOSE-6-PHOSPHATE DEHYDROGENASE (G6PD) DEFICIENCY
A. X-linked recessive disorder resulting in reduced half-life of G6PD; renders cells susceptible to oxidative stress
   1. RBCs are normally exposed to oxidative stress, in particular H_2O_2.
   2. Glutathione (an antioxidant) neutralizes H_2O_2, but becomes oxidized in the process.
   3. NADPH, a by-product of G6PD, is needed to regenerate reduced glutathione.
   4. ↓ G6PD → ↓ NADPH → ↓ reduced glutathione → oxidative injury by H_2O_2 → intravascular hemolysis
B. G6PD deficiency has two major variants.
   1. African variant—mildly reduced half-life of G6PD leading to mild intravascular hemolysis with oxidative stress
   2. Mediterranean variant—markedly reduced half-life of G6PD leading to marked intravascular hemolysis with oxidative stress
   3. High carrier frequency in both populations is likely due to protective role against falciparum malaria.

    C. Oxidative stress precipitates Hb as Heinz bodies.
        1. Causes of oxidative stress include infections, drugs (e.g., primaquine, sulfa drugs, and dapsone), and fava beans.
        2. Heinz bodies are removed from RBCs by splenic macrophages, resulting in bite cells (Fig. 5.11).
        3. Leads to predominantly intravascular hemolysis
    D. Presents with hemoglobinuria and back pain hours after exposure to oxidative stress
    E. Heinz preparation is used to screen for disease (precipitated hemoglobin can only be seen with a special Heinz stain, Fig. 5.12); enzyme studies confirm deficiency (performed weeks after hemolytic episode resolves).

III. **IMMUNE HEMOLYTIC ANEMIA (IHA)**
    A. Antibody-mediated (IgG or IgM) destruction of RBCs
    B. IgG-mediated disease usually involves extravascular hemolysis.
        1. IgG binds RBCs in the relatively warm temperature of the central body (warm agglutinin); membrane of antibody-coated RBC is consumed by splenic macrophages, resulting in spherocytes.
        2. Associated with SLE (most common cause), CLL, and certain drugs (classically, penicillin and cephalosporins)
            i. Drug may attach to RBC membrane (e.g., penicillin) with subsequent binding of antibody to drug-membrane complex
            ii. Drug may induce production of autoantibodies (e.g., α-methyldopa) that bind self antigens on RBCs
        3. Treatment involves cessation of the offending drug, steroids, IVIG, and, if necessary, splenectomy.
    C. IgM-mediated disease usually involves intravascular hemolysis.
        1. IgM binds RBCs and fixes complement in the relatively cold temperature of the extremities (cold agglutinin). ⤷ MAC
        2. Associated with *Mycoplasma pneumoniae* and infectious mononucleosis
    D. Coombs test is used to diagnose IHA; testing can be direct or indirect.
        1. Direct Coombs test confirms the presence of antibody-coated RBCs. Anti-IgG is added to patient RBCs; agglutination occurs if RBCs are already coated with antibody. This is the most important test for IHA.
        2. Indirect Coombs test confirms the presence of antibodies in patient serum. Anti-IgG and test RBCs are mixed with the patient serum; agglutination occurs if serum antibodies are present.

IV. **MICROANGIOPATHIC HEMOLYTIC ANEMIA**
    A. Intravascular hemolysis that results from vascular pathology; RBCs are destroyed as they pass through the circulation.

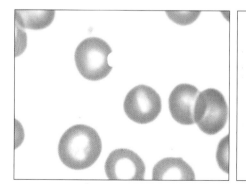

Fig. 5.11 Bite cell.

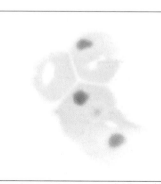

Fig. 5.12 Heinz bodies (Heinz preparation).

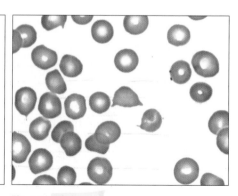

Fig. 5.13 Schistocyte.

1. Iron deficiency anemia occurs with chronic hemolysis.
B. Occurs with microthrombi (TTP-HUS, DIC, HELLP), prosthetic heart valves, and aortic stenosis; when present, microthrombi produce schistocytes on blood smear (Fig. 5.13).

V. MALARIA
A. Infection of RBCs and liver with *Plasmodium* (Fig. 5.14); transmitted by the female *Anopheles* mosquito
B. RBCs rupture as a part of the *Plasmodium* life cycle, resulting in intravascular hemolysis and cyclical fever.
   1. *P falciparum*—daily fever
   2. *P vivax* and *P ovale*—fever every other day
C. Spleen also consumes some infected RBCs; results in mild extravascular hemolysis with splenomegaly

ANEMIA DUE TO UNDERPRODUCTION
I. BASIC PRINCIPLES
A. Decreased production of RBCs by bone marrow; characterized by low corrected reticulocyte count
B. Etiologies include
   1. Causes of microcytic and macrocytic anemia
   2. Renal failure—decreased production of EPO by peritubular interstitial cells
   3. Damage to bone marrow precursor cells (may result in anemia or pancytopenia)

II. PARVOVIRUS B19
A. Infects progenitor red cells and temporarily halts erythropoiesis; leads to significant anemia in the setting of preexisting marrow stress (e.g., sickle cell anemia).
B. Treatment is supportive (infection is self-limited).

III. APLASTIC ANEMIA
A. Damage to hematopoietic stem cells, resulting in pancytopenia (anemia, thrombocytopenia, and leukopenia) with low reticulocyte count
B. Etiologies include drugs or chemicals, viral infections, and autoimmune damage.
C. Biopsy reveals an empty, fatty marrow (Fig. 5.15).
D. Treatment includes cessation of any causative drugs and supportive care with transfusions and marrow-stimulating factors (e.g., erythropoietin, GM-CSF, and G-CSF).
   1. Immunosuppression may be helpful as some idiopathic cases are due to abnormal T-cell activation with release of cytokines.

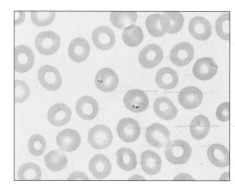 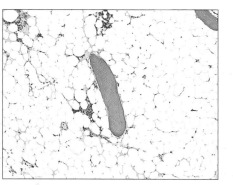

Fig. 5.14 Erythrocytes infected with *P falciparum*. **Fig. 5.15** Aplastic anemia. (Courtesy of Paulo Mourao, MD)

2. May require bone marrow transplantation as a last resort

IV. MYELOPHTHISIC PROCESS

A. Pathologic process (e.g., metastatic cancer) that replaces bone marrow; hematopoiesis is impaired, resulting in pancytopenia.

White Blood Cell Disorders

6

LEUKOPENIA AND LEUKOCYTOSIS

I. **BASIC PRINCIPLES**

A. Hematopoiesis occurs via a stepwise maturation of CD34$^+$ hematopoietic stem cells (Fig. 6.1).

B. Cells mature and are released from the bone marrow into the blood.

C. A normal white blood cell (WBC) count is approximately 5–10 K/μL.

1. A low WBC count (< 5 K) is called leukopenia.

2. A high WBC count (> 10 K) is called leukocytosis.

3. A low or high WBC count is usually due to a decrease or increase in one particular cell lineage.

II. **LEUKOPENIA**

A. Neutropenia refers to a decreased number of circulating neutrophils. Causes include

1. Drug toxicity (e.g., chemotherapy with alkylating agents)—Damage to stem cells results in decreased production of WBCs, especially neutrophils.

2. Severe infection (e.g., gram-negative sepsis)—Increased movement of neutrophils into tissues results in decreased circulating neutrophils.

3. As a treatment, GM-CSF or G-CSF may be used to boost granulocyte production, thereby decreasing risk of infection in neutropenic.

B. Lymphopenia refers to a decreased number of circulating lymphocytes. Causes include

1. Immunodeficiency (e.g., DiGeorge syndrome or HIV)

2. High cortisol state (e.g., exogenous corticosteroids or Cushing syndrome)—induces apoptosis of lymphocytes

3. Autoimmune destruction (e.g., systemic lupus erythematosus)

4. Whole body radiation—Lymphocytes are highly sensitive to radiation; lymphopenia is the earliest change to emerge after whole body radiation.

III. **LEUKOCYTOSIS**

A. Neutrophilic leukocytosis refers to increased circulating neutrophils. Causes include

1. Bacterial infection or tissue necrosis—induces release of marginated pool and bone marrow neutrophils, including immature forms (left shift); immature cells are characterized by decreased Fc receptors (CD16).

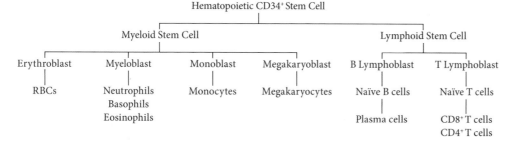

Fig. 6.1 Hematopoiesis.

2. High cortisol state—impairs leukocyte adhesion, leading to release of marginated pool of neutrophils – *neutrophils that hang on vessels*

B. Monocytosis refers to increased circulating monocytes. Causes include chronic inflammatory states (e.g., autoimmune and infectious) and malignancy.

C. Eosinophilia refers to increased circulating eosinophils. Causes include allergic reactions (type I hypersensitivity), parasitic infections, and Hodgkin lymphoma. Eosinophilia is driven by increased eosinophil chemotactic factor. *(IL-5)*

D. Basophilia refers to increased circulating basophils; classically seen in chronic myeloid leukemia

E. Lymphocytic leukocytosis refers to increased circulating lymphocytes. Causes include

1. Viral infections—T lymphocytes undergo hyperplasia in response to virally infected cells.

2. *Bordetella pertussis* infection—Bacteria produce lymphocytosis-promoting factor, which blocks circulating lymphocytes from leaving the blood to enter the lymph node.

IV. INFECTIOUS MONONUCLEOSIS (IM)

A. EBV infection that results in a lymphocytic leukocytosis comprised of reactive CD8$^+$ T cells; CMV is a less common cause.

1. EBV is transmitted by saliva ("kissing disease"); classically affects teenagers

B. EBV primarily infects

1. Oropharynx, resulting in pharyngitis

2. Liver, resulting in hepatitis with hepatomegaly and elevated liver enzymes

3. B cells

C. CD8$^+$ T-cell response leads to

1. Generalized lymphadenopathy (LAD) due to T-cell hyperplasia in the lymph node paracortex

2. Splenomegaly due to T-cell hyperplasia in the periarterial lymphatic sheath (PALS)

3. High WBC count with atypical lymphocytes (reactive CD8$^+$ T cells) in the blood (Fig. 6.2) *↳large nucleus lots of blue cytosol*

D. The monospot test is used for screening.

1. Detects IgM antibodies that cross-react with horse or sheep red blood cells (heterophile antibodies)

2. Usually turns positive within 1 week after infection

3. A negative monospot test suggests CMV as a possible cause of IM.

4. Definitive diagnosis is made by serologic testing for the EBV viral capsid antigen.

Lymph node

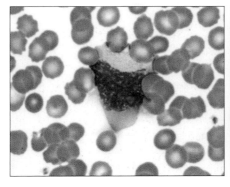

Fig. 6.2 Atypical lymphocyte, infectious mononucleosis.

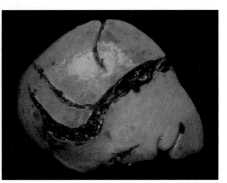

Fig. 6.3 Splenic rupture. (Courtesy of K.V. Santosh, MD)

E. Complications
1. Increased risk for splenic rupture (Fig. 6.3); patients are generally advised to avoid contact sports for one month.
2. Rash if exposed to ampicillin
3. Dormancy of virus in B cells leads to increased risk for both recurrence and B-cell lymphoma, especially if immunodeficiency (e.g., HIV) develops.

ACUTE LEUKEMIA

I. **BASIC PRINCIPLES**
A. Neoplastic proliferation of blasts; defined as the accumulation of > 20% blasts in the bone marrow.
B. Increased blasts "crowd-out" normal hematopoiesis, resulting in an "acute" presentation with anemia (fatigue), thrombocytopenia (bleeding), or neutropenia (infection).
C. Blasts usually enter the blood stream, resulting in a high WBC count.
1. Blasts are large, immature cells, often with punched out nucleoli (Fig. 6.4).
D. Acute leukemia is subdivided into acute lymphoblastic leukemia (ALL) or acute myelogenous leukemia (AML) based on the phenotype of the blasts.

II. **ACUTE LYMPHOBLASTIC LEUKEMIA**
A. Neoplastic accumulation of lymphoblasts (> 20%) in the bone marrow
1. Lymphoblasts are characterized by positive nuclear staining for TdT, a DNA polymerase.
2. TdT is absent in myeloid blasts and mature lymphocytes.
B. Most commonly arises in children; associated with Down syndrome (usually arises *after* the age of 5 years)
C. Subclassified into B-ALL and T-ALL based on surface markers.
D. B-ALL is the most common type of ALL.
1. Usually characterized by lymphoblasts (TdT+) that express CD10, CD19, and CD20.
2. Excellent response to chemotherapy; requires prophylaxis to scrotum and CSF (Fig. 6.5)
3. Prognosis is based on cytogenetic abnormalities.
   translocation i. t(12;21) has a good prognosis; more commonly seen in children
   ii. t(9;22) has a poor prognosis; more commonly seen in adults (Philadelphia+ ALL)
E. T-ALL is characterized by lymphoblasts (TdT+) that express markers ranging from CD2 to CD8 (e.g., CD3, CD4, CD7). The blasts do not express CD10.

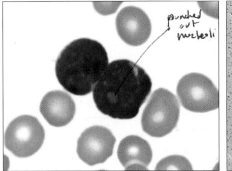

punched out nucleoli

Fig. 6.4 Blasts of acute leukemia.

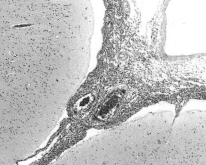

Fig. 6.5 Acute lymphoblastic leukemia involving meninges.

T-ALL
thymic blast
teenager

1. Usually presents in teenagers as a mediastinal (thymic) mass (called acute lymphoblastic lymph*oma* because the malignant cells form a mass)

III. ACUTE MYELOID LEUKEMIA

A. Neoplastic accumulation of immature myeloid cells (> 20%) in the bone marrow

B. Myeloblasts are usually characterized by positive cytoplasmic staining for myeloperoxidase (MPO).

    1. Crystal aggregates of MPO may be seen as Auer rods (Fig. 6.6).

C. Most commonly arises in older adults (average age is 50–60 years)

D. Subclassified based on cytogenetic abnormalities, lineage of myeloblasts, and surface markers. High-yield subtypes include

    1. Acute promyelocytic leukemia (APL)

        i. Characterized by t(15;17), which involves translocation of the retinoic acid receptor (RAR) on chromosome 17 to chromosome 15; RAR disruption blocks maturation and promyelocytes (blasts) accumulate.

        ii. Abnormal promyelocytes contain numerous primary granules that increase the risk for DIC.

        iii. Treatment is with all-*trans*-retinoic acid (ATRA, a vitamin A derivative), which binds the altered receptor and causes the blasts to mature (and eventually die).

    2. Acute monocytic leukemia

        i. Proliferation of monoblasts; usually lack MPO

        ii. Blasts characteristically infiltrate gums (Fig. 6.7).

    3. Acute megakaryoblastic leukemia

        i. Proliferation of megakaryoblasts; lack MPO

        ii. Associated with Down syndrome (usually arises *before* the age of 5)

E. AML may also arise from pre-existing dysplasia (myelodysplastic syndromes), especially with prior exposure to alkylating agents or radiotherapy.

    1. Myelodysplastic syndromes usually present with cytopenias, hypercellular bone marrow, abnormal maturation of cells, and increased blasts (< 20%).

    2. Most patients die from infection or bleeding, though some progress to acute leukemia.

CHRONIC LEUKEMIA

I. BASIC PRINCIPLES

A. Neoplastic proliferation of mature circulating lymphocytes; characterized by a high WBC count

B. Usually insidious in onset and seen in older adults

smudge cell = CLL

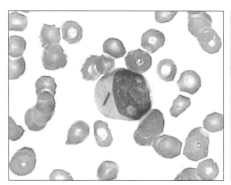

Fig. 6.6 Acute myelogenous leukemia with Auer rod. (Courtesy of Paulo Mourao, MD)

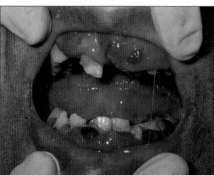

Fig. 6.7 Acute monocytic leukemia. (Courtesy of Drs. H. Fred and H. van Dijk, *Images of Memorable Cases*)

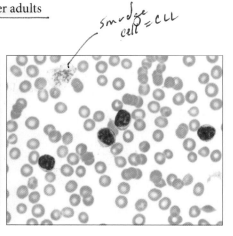

Fig. 6.8 Chronic lymphocytic leukemia.

II. CHRONIC LYMPHOCYTIC LEUKEMIA (CLL)

A. Neoplastic proliferation of naïve B cells that co-express CD5 and CD20; most common leukemia overall

B. Increased lymphocytes and smudge cells are seen on blood smear (Fig. 6.8).

C. Involvement of lymph nodes leads to generalized lymphadenopathy and is called small lymphocytic lymphoma.

D. Complications include

  1. Hypogammaglobulinemia—Infection is the most common cause of death in CLL.

  2. Autoimmune hemolytic anemia

  3. Transformation to diffuse large B-cell lymphoma (Richter transformation)—marked clinically by an enlarging lymph node or spleen

III. HAIRY CELL LEUKEMIA

A. Neoplastic proliferation of mature B cells characterized by hairy cytoplasmic processes (Fig. 6.9)

B. Cells are positive for tartrate-resistant acid phosphatase (TRAP). *TRAPPED in bone marrow*

C. Clinical features include splenomegaly (due to accumulation of hairy cells in red pulp) and "dry tap" on bone marrow aspiration (due to marrow fibrosis). Lymphadenopathy is usually absent.

D. Excellent response to 2-CDA (cladribine), an adenosine deaminase inhibitor; adenosine accumulates to toxic levels in neoplastic B cells. *→ Purine degradation pathway*

IV. ADULT T-CELL LEUKEMIA/LYMPHOMA (ATLL)

A. Neoplastic proliferation of mature CD4+ T cells

B. Associated with HTLV-1; most commonly seen in Japan and the Caribbean

C. Clinical features include rash (skin infiltration), generalized lymphadenopathy with hepatosplenomegaly, and lytic (punched-out) bone lesions with hypercalcemia.

V. MYCOSIS FUNGOIDES

A. Neoplastic proliferation of mature CD4+ T cells that infiltrate the skin, producing localized skin rash, plaques, and nodules. Aggregates of neoplastic cells in the epidermis are called Pautrier microabscesses.

B. Cells can spread to involve the blood, producing Sezary syndrome.

  1. Characteristic lymphocytes with cerebriform nuclei (Sezary cells) are seen on blood smear (Fig. 6.10).

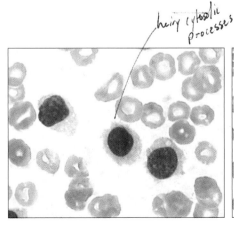

hairy cytoplasmic processes

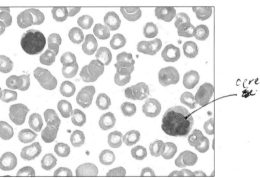

cerebriform nuclei

Fig. 6.9 Hairy cell leukemia. (Courtesy of Paulo Mourao, MD)

Fig. 6.10 Sezary cells. (Courtesy of Paulo Mourao, MD)

MYELOPROLIFERATIVE DISORDERS (MPD)

AML
ALL
CL
MPD

I. **BASIC PRINCIPLES**
   A. Neoplastic proliferation of mature cells of myeloid lineage; disease of late adulthood (average age is 50–60 years)
   B. Results in high WBC count with hypercellular bone marrow
      1. Cells of all myeloid lineages are increased; classified based on the dominant myeloid cell produced
   C. Complications include
      1. Increased risk for hyperuricemia and gout due to high turnover of cells
      2. Progression to marrow fibrosis or transformation to acute leukemia

II. **CHRONIC MYELOID LEUKEMIA (CML)**
   A. Neoplastic proliferation of mature myeloid cells, especially granulocytes and their precursors; basophils are characteristically increased (Fig. 6.11).
   B. Driven by t(9;22) (Philadelphia chromosome) which generates a BCR-ABL fusion protein with increased tyrosine kinase activity.
      1. First line treatment is imatinib, which blocks tyrosine kinase activity.
   C. Splenomegaly is common. Enlarging spleen suggests progression to accelerated phase of disease; transformation to acute leukemia usually follows shortly thereafter.
      1. Can transform to AML (2/3 of cases) or ALL (1/3 of cases) since mutation is in a pluripotent stem cell. *(HSC)*
   D. CML is distinguished from a leukemoid reaction (reactive neutrophilic leukocytosis) by *↳?in response to infection*
      1. Negative leukocyte alkaline phosphatase (LAP) stain (granulocytes in a leukemoid reaction are LAP positive)
      2. Increased basophils (absent with leukemoid reaction)
      3. t(9;22) (absent in leukemoid reaction)

III. **POLYCYTHEMIA VERA (PV)**
   A. Neoplastic proliferation of mature myeloid cells, especially RBCs
      1. Granulocytes and platelets are also increased.
   B. Associated with JAK2 kinase mutation
   C. Clinical symptoms are mostly due to hyperviscosity of blood.
      1. Blurry vision and headache
      2. Increased risk of venous thrombosis (e.g., hepatic vein, portal vein, and dural sinus)   ↳   *↳Budd-Chiari syndrome*
      3. Flushed face due to congestion (plethora)
      4. Itching, especially after bathing (due to histamine release from increased mast cells)
   D. Treatment is phlebotomy; second-line therapy is hydroxyurea.

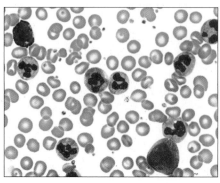

Fig. 6.11 Chronic myelogenous leukemia.

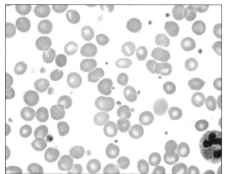

Fig. 6.12 Essential thrombocythemia.

1. Without treatment, death usually occurs within one year.
   E. PV must be distinguished from reactive polycythemia.
   1. In PV, erythropoietin (EPO) levels are decreased, and Sao$_2$ is normal.
   2. In reactive polycythemia due to high altitude or lung disease, Sao$_2$ is low, and EPO is increased.
   3. In reactive polycythemia due to ectopic EPO production from renal cell carcinoma, EPO is high, and Sao$_2$ is normal.

IV. ESSENTIAL THROMBOCYTHEMIA (ET)

A. Neoplastic proliferation of mature myeloid cells, especially platelets (Fig. 6.12)
   1. RBCs and granulocytes are also increased.
B. Associated with JAK2 kinase mutation
C. Symptoms are related to an increased risk of bleeding and/or thrombosis.
   1. Rarely progresses to marrow fibrosis or acute leukemia
   2. No significant risk for hyperuricemia or gout

V. MYELOFIBROSIS

A. Neoplastic proliferation of mature myeloid cells, especially megakaryocytes
   1. Associated with JAK2 kinase mutation (50% of cases)
B. Megakaryocytes produce excess platelet-derived growth factor (PDGF) causing marrow fibrosis (Fig. 6.13).
C. Clinical features include
   1. Splenomegaly due to extramedullary hematopoiesis
   2. Leukoerythroblastic smear (tear-drop RBCs, nucleated RBCs, and immature granulocytes, Fig. 6.14)
   3. Increased risk of infection, thrombosis, and bleeding *b/c extramedullary hematopoiesis doesn't produce enough*

reticulin gates in bone marrow inhibit immature cells from leaving

LYMPHADENOPATHY (LAD)

I. BASIC PRINCIPLES

A. LAD refers to enlarged lymph nodes.
   1. Painful LAD is usually seen in lymph nodes that are draining a region of acute infection (acute lymphadenitis).
   2. Painless LAD can be seen with chronic inflammation (chronic lymphadenitis), metastatic carcinoma, or lymphoma.
B. In inflammation, lymph node enlargement is due to hyperplasia of particular regions of the lymph node (Fig. 6.15).
   1. Follicular hyperplasia (B-cell region) is seen with rheumatoid arthritis and early stages of HIV infection, for example.

↳CD4⁺ cells - follicular dendritic

collagen in marrow space

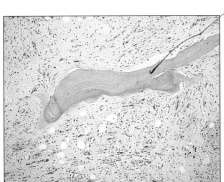

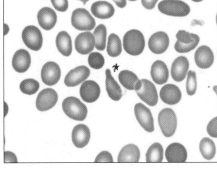

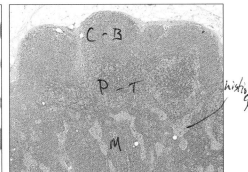

Fig. 6.13 Myelofibrosis.   **Fig. 6.14** Tear-drop RBC.   **Fig. 6.15** Normal lymph node.

2. Paracortex hyperplasia (T-cell region) is seen with viral infections (e.g., infectious mononucleosis).
3. Hyperplasia of sinus histiocytes is seen in lymph nodes that are draining a tissue with cancer.

LYMPHOMA

I. **BASIC PRINCIPLES**
   A. Neoplastic proliferation of lymphoid cells that forms a mass; may arise in a lymph node or in extranodal tissue
   B. Divided into non-Hodgkin lymphoma (NHL, 60%) and Hodgkin lymphoma (HL, 40%) (Table 6.1)
   C. NHL is further classified based on cell type (e.g., B versus T), cell size, pattern of cell growth, expression of surface markers, and cytogenetic translocations.
     1. Small B cells—follicular lymphoma, mantle cell lymphoma, marginal zone lymphoma, and small lymphocytic lymphoma (i.e., CLL cells that involve tissue)
     2. Intermediate-sized B cells—Burkitt lymphoma
     3. Large B cells—diffuse large B-cell lymphoma

[Handwritten margin notes: Cortex - B cells - follicle - somatic hypermutation - mantle - margin ; Size ; Classification]

Table 6.1: Differences Between Non-Hodgkin Lymphoma and Hodgkin Lymphoma

	NON-HODGKIN LYMPHOMA	HODGKIN LYMPHOMA
Overall frequency	60%	40%
Malignant cells	Lymphoid cells	Reed-Sternberg cells
Composition of mass	Lymphoid cells	Predominantly reactive cells (inflammatory cells and fibrosis)
Clinical	Painless lymphadenopathy, usually arises in late adulthood	Painless lymphadenopathy occasionally with 'B' symptoms, usually arises in young adults
Spread	Diffuse; often extranodal	Contiguous; rarely extranodal
Staging	Limited importance	Guides therapy; radiation is the mainstay of treatment.
Leukemic phase	Occurs	Does not occur

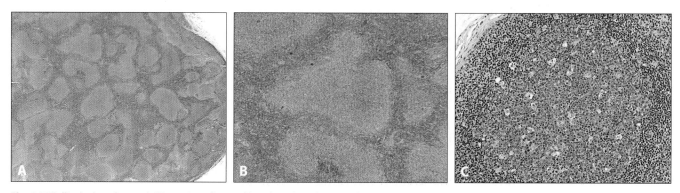

Fig. 6.16 Follicular lymphoma. **A,** Disruption of normal lymph node architecture by neoplastic follicles. **B,** Neoplastic follicles lacking tingible body macrophages. **C,** Reactive follicular hyperplasia with tingible body macrophages for comparison.

II. FOLLICULAR LYMPHOMA

A. Neoplastic proliferation of small B cells (CD20⁺) that form follicle-like nodules (Fig. 6.16A)

B. Presents in late adulthood with painless lymphadenopathy

C. Driven by t(14;18)

   1. *BCL2* on chromosome 18 translocates to the Ig heavy chain locus on chromosome 14. *[handwritten: → stabilizes mitochondrial membrane]*

   2. Results in overexpression of Bcl2, which inhibits apoptosis

D. Treatment is reserved for patients who are symptomatic and involves low-dose chemotherapy or rituximab (anti-CD20 antibody).

E. Progression to diffuse large B-cell lymphoma is an important complication; presents as an enlarging lymph node

F. Follicular lymphoma is distinguished from reactive follicular hyperplasia by

   1. Disruption of normal lymph node architecture (maintained in follicular hyperplasia)

   2. Lack of tingible body macrophages in germinal centers (tingible body macrophages are present in follicular hyperplasia, Fig. 6.16B,C)

   3. Bcl2 expression in follicles (not expressed in follicular hyperplasia)

   4. Monoclonality (follicular hyperplasia is polyclonal)

[handwritten margin note: tingible body macrophages clean up apoptotic debris]

III. MANTLE CELL LYMPHOMA

A. Neoplastic proliferation of small B cells (CD20⁺) that expands the mantle zone

B. Presents in late adulthood with painless lymphadenopathy

C. Driven by t(11;14)

   1. Cyclin D1 gene on chromosome 11 translocates to Ig heavy chain locus on chromosome 14. *[handwritten: → phosphorylates]*

   2. Overexpression of cyclin D1 promotes G1/S transition in the cell cycle, facilitating neoplastic proliferation.

IV. MARGINAL ZONE LYMPHOMA

A. Neoplastic proliferation of small B cells (CD20⁺) that expands the marginal zone

B. Associated with chronic inflammatory states such as Hashimoto thyroiditis, Sjögren syndrome, and *H pylori* gastritis

   1. The marginal zone is formed by post-germinal center B cells.

C. MALToma is marginal zone lymphoma in mucosal sites.

   1. Gastric MALToma may regress with treatment of *H Pylori*.

V. BURKITT LYMPHOMA

A. Neoplastic proliferation of intermediate-sized B cells (CD20⁺); associated with EBV

B. Classically presents as an extranodal mass in a child or young adult

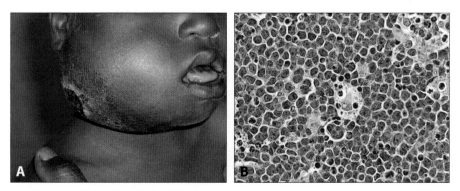

Fig. 6.17 Burkitt lymphoma. **A**, Involvement of jaw. **B**, 'Starry-sky' appearance. (A, Courtesy Mike Blyth)

    1. African form usually involves the jaw (Fig. 6.17A).

    2. Sporadic form usually involves the abdomen.

  C. Driven by translocations of *c-myc* (chromosome 8)

    1. t(8;14) is most common, resulting in translocation of *c-myc* to the Ig heavy chain locus on chromosome 14.

    2. Overexpression of *c-myc* oncogene promotes cell growth.

  D. Characterized by high mitotic index and 'starry-sky' appearance on microscopy (Fig. 6.17B)

VI. **DIFFUSE LARGE B-CELL LYMPHOMA**

  A. Neoplastic proliferation of large B cells (CD20$^+$) that grow diffusely in sheets

    1. Most common form of NHL

    2. Clinically aggressive (high-grade)

  B. Arises sporadically or from transformation of a low-grade lymphoma (e.g., follicular lymphoma)

    1. Presents in late adulthood as an enlarging lymph node or an extranodal mass

HODGKIN LYMPHOMA (HL)

I. **BASIC PRINCIPLES**

  A. Neoplastic proliferation of Reed-Sternberg (RS) cells, which are large B cells with multilobed nuclei and prominent nucleoli ('owl-eyed nuclei', Fig. 6.18); classically positive for CD15 and CD30

  B. RS cells secrete cytokines.

    1. Occasionally results in 'B' symptoms (fever, chills, weight loss, and night sweats)

    2. Attract reactive lymphocytes, plasma cells, macrophages, and eosinophils

    3. May lead to fibrosis

  C. Reactive inflammatory cells make up a bulk of the tumor and form the basis for classification of HL. Subtypes include

    1. Nodular sclerosis

    2. Lymphocyte-rich

    3. Mixed cellularity

    4. Lymphocyte-depleted

  D. Nodular sclerosis is the most common subtype of HL (70% of all cases).

    1. Classic presentation is an enlarging cervical or mediastinal lymph node in a young adult, usually female.

    2. Lymph node is divided by bands of sclerosis (Fig. 6.19A); RS cells are present in lake-like spaces (lacunar cells, Fig. 6.19B).

  E. Important considerations regarding other subtypes of HL

    1. Lymphocyte-rich has the best prognosis of all types.

Sclerosis = hard

Reed-Sternberg

lacunar cells

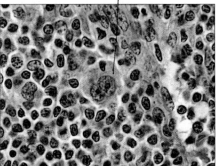

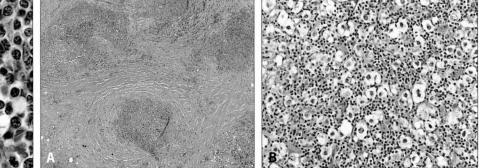

Fig. 6.18 Reed-Sternberg cell.

Fig. 6.19 Hodgkin lymphoma, nodular sclerosis type. **A**, Sclerosis of lymph node. **B**, Reed-Sternberg cells in lacunar spaces.

2. Mixed cellularity is often associated with abundant eosinophils (RS cells produce IL-5).

3. Lymphocyte-depleted is the most aggressive of all types; usually seen in the elderly and HIV-positive individuals

PLASMA CELL DISORDERS (DYSCRASIAS)

I. **MULTIPLE MYELOMA** ← disorder

A. Malignant proliferation of plasma cells in the bone marrow

1. Most common primary malignancy of bone; metastatic cancer, however, is the most common malignant lesion of bone overall.

2. High serum IL-6 may be present; stimulates plasma cell growth and immunoglobulin production

B. Clinical features include

1. Bone pain with hypercalcemia—Neoplastic plasma cells activate the RANK *via osteoclast activation factor* receptor on osteoclasts, leading to bone destruction. Lytic, 'punched-out' skeletal lesions are seen on x-ray (Fig. 6.20A), especially in the vertebrae and skull; increased risk for fracture

2. Elevated serum protein—Neoplastic plasma cells produce immunoglobulin; M spike is present on serum protein electrophoresis (SPEP), most commonly due to monoclonal IgG or IgA. *M spike = monoclonal Ab*

3. Increased risk of infection—Monoclonal antibody lacks antigenic diversity; infection is the most common cause of death in multiple myeloma.

4. Rouleaux formation of RBCs on blood smear—Increased serum protein decreases charge between RBCs (Fig. 6.20B).

5. Primary AL amyloidosis—Free light chains circulate in serum and deposit in tissues.

6. Proteinuria—Free light chain is excreted in the urine as Bence Jones protein; deposition in kidney tubules leads to risk for renal failure (myeloma kidney).

II. **MONOCLONAL GAMMOPATHY OF UNDETERMINED SIGNIFICANCE (MGUS)**

A. Increased serum protein with M spike on SPEP; other features of multiple myeloma are absent (e.g., no lytic bone lesions, hypercalcemia, AL amyloid, or Bence Jones proteinuria).

B. Common in elderly (seen in 5% of 70-year-old individuals); 1% of patients with MGUS develop multiple myeloma each year.

III. **WALDENSTRÖM MACROGLOBULINEMIA**

A. B-cell lymphoma with monoclonal IgM production

B. Clinical features include

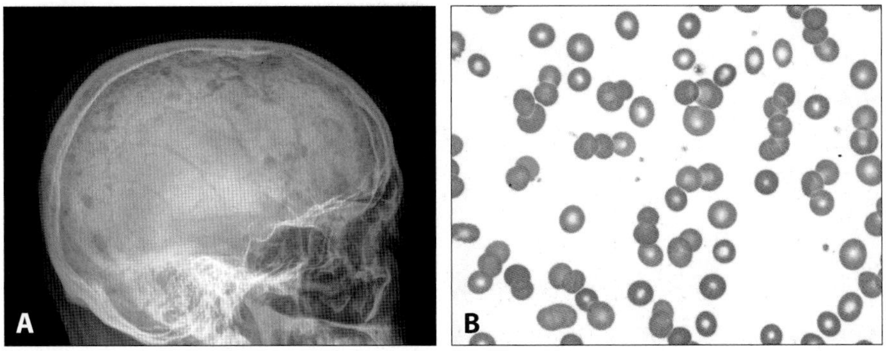

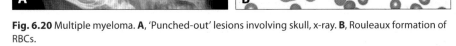

Fig. 6.20 Multiple myeloma. **A**, 'Punched-out' lesions involving skull, x-ray. **B**, Rouleaux formation of RBCs. **Fig. 6.21** Birbeck granule, electron microscopy. (Courtesy of humpath.com)

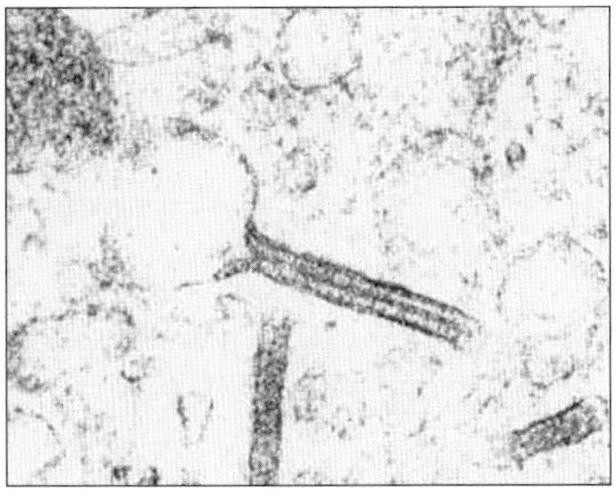

1. Generalized lymphadenopathy; lytic bone lesions are absent.
2. Increased serum protein with M spike (comprised of IgM)
3. Visual and neurologic deficits (e.g., retinal hemorrhage or stroke)—IgM (large pentamer) causes serum hyperviscosity.
4. Bleeding—Viscous serum results in defective platelet aggregation.

C. Acute complications are treated with plasmapheresis, which removes IgM from the serum.

LANGERHANS CELL HISTIOCYTOSIS

I. **BASIC PRINCIPLES**

A. Langerhans cells are specialized dendritic cells found predominantly in the skin.
1. Derived from bone marrow monocytes
2. Present antigen to naïve T cells

B. Langerhans cell histiocytosis is a neoplastic proliferation of Langerhans cells.
1. Characteristic Birbeck (tennis racket) granules are seen on electron microscopy (Fig. 6.21); cells are CD1a$^+$ and S100$^+$ by immunohistochemistry.

II. **LETTERER-SIWE DISEASE**

A. Malignant proliferation of Langerhans cells
B. Classic presentation is skin rash and cystic skeletal defects in an infant (< 2 years old).
C. Multiple organs may be involved; rapidly fatal

III. **EOSINOPHILIC GRANULOMA**

A. Benign proliferation of Langerhans cells in bone
B. Classic presentation is pathologic fracture in an adolescent; skin is not involved.
C. Biopsy shows Langerhans cells with mixed inflammatory cells, including numerous eosinophils.

IV. **HAND-SCHÜLLER-CHRISTIAN DISEASE**

A. Malignant proliferation of Langerhans cells
B. Classic presentation is scalp rash, lytic skull defects, diabetes insipidus, and exophthalmos in a child.

Vascular Pathology

7

VASCULITIS

I. **BASIC PRINCIPLES**
   A. Inflammation of the blood vessel wall
      1. Arterial wall is comprised of three layers: endothelial intima, smooth muscle media, and connective tissue adventitia (Fig. 7.1).
   B. Etiology is usually unknown; most cases are not infectious.
   C. Clinical features include
      1. Nonspecific symptoms of inflammation (e.g., fever, fatigue, weight loss, and myalgias)
      2. Symptoms of organ ischemia—due to luminal narrowing or thrombosis of the inflamed vessels
   D. Divided into large-, medium-, and small-vessel vasculitides
      1. Large-vessel vasculitis involves the aorta and its major branches.
      2. Medium-vessel vasculitis involves muscular arteries that supply organs.
      3. Small-vessel vasculitis involves arterioles, capillaries, and venules.

II. **LARGE-VESSEL VASCULITIS**
   A. Temporal (Giant Cell) Arteritis
      1. Granulomatous vasculitis that classically involves branches of the carotid artery
      2. Most common form of vasculitis in older adults (> 50 years); usually affects females
      3. Presents as headache (temporal artery involvement), visual disturbances (ophthalmic artery involvement), and jaw claudication. Flu-like symptoms with joint and muscle pain (polymyalgia rheumatica) are often present. ESR is elevated.
      4. Biopsy reveals inflamed vessel wall with giant cells and intimal fibrosis (Fig. 7.2).
         i. Lesions are segmental; diagnosis requires biopsy of a long segment of vessel, and a negative biopsy does not exclude disease.
      5. Treatment is corticosteroids; high risk of blindness without treatment
   B. Takayasu Arteritis
      1. Granulomatous vasculitis that classically involves the aortic arch at branch points
      2. Presents in adults < 50 years old (classically, young Asian females) as visual and neurologic symptoms with a weak or absent pulse in the upper extremity ('pulseless disease'). ESR is elevated.
      3. Treatment is corticosteroids.

III. **MEDIUM-VESSEL VASCULITIS**
   A. Polyarteritis Nodosa
      1. Necrotizing vasculitis involving multiple organs; lungs are spared.
      2. Classically presents in young adults as hypertension (renal artery involvement), abdominal pain with melena (mesenteric artery involvement), neurologic disturbances, and skin lesions. Associated with serum HBsAg

3. Lesions of varying stages are present. Early lesion consists of transmural inflammation with fibrinoid necrosis (Fig. 7.3); eventually heals with fibrosis, producing a 'string-of-pearls' appearance on imaging

4. Treatment is corticosteroids and cyclophosphamide; fatal if not treated

B. Kawasaki Disease

1. Classically affects Asian children < 4 years old

2. Presents with nonspecific signs including fever, conjunctivitis, erythematous rash of palms and soles, and enlarged cervical lymph nodes

3. Coronary artery involvement is common and leads to risk for (1) thrombosis with myocardial infarction and (2) aneurysm with rupture.

4. Treatment is aspirin and IVIG; disease is self-limited.

C. Buerger Disease

1. Necrotizing vasculitis involving digits

2. Presents with ulceration, gangrene, and autoamputation of fingers and toes; Raynaud phenomenon is often present.

3. Highly associated with heavy smoking; treatment is smoking cessation.

IV. **SMALL-VESSEL VASCULITIS**

A. Wegener Granulomatosis

1. Necrotizing granulomatous vasculitis involving nasopharynx, lungs, and kidneys

2. Classic presentation is a middle-aged male with sinusitis or nasopharyngeal ulceration, hemoptysis with bilateral nodular lung infiltrates, and hematuria due to rapidly progressive glomerulonephritis.

3. Serum c-ANCA levels correlate with disease activity.

4. Biopsy reveals large necrotizing granulomas with adjacent necrotizing vasculitis (Fig. 7.4).

5. Treatment is cyclophosphamide and steroids; relapses are common.

B. Microscopic Polyangiitis

1. Necrotizing vasculitis involving multiple organs, especially lung and kidney

2. Presentation is similar to Wegener granulomatosis, but nasopharyngeal involvement and granulomas are absent.

3. Serum p-ANCA levels correlate with disease activity.

4. Treatment is corticosteroids and cyclophosphamide; relapses are common.

C. Churg-Strauss Syndrome

1. Necrotizing granulomatous inflammation with eosinophils involving multiple organs, especially lungs and heart

2. Asthma and peripheral eosinophilia are often present.

3. Serum p-ANCA levels correlate with disease activity.

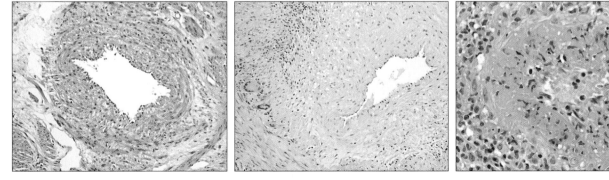

Fig. 7.1 Normal muscular artery.   **Fig. 7.2** Temporal (giant cell) arteritis.   **Fig. 7.3** Fibrinoid necrosis, polyarteritis nodosa.

D. Henoch-Schönlein Purpura
1. Vasculitis due to IgA immune complex deposition; most common vasculitis in children
2. Presents with palpable purpura on buttocks and legs, GI pain and bleeding, and hematuria (IgA nephropathy); usually occurs following an upper respiratory tract infection
3. Disease is self-limited, but may recur; treated with steroids, if severe

HYPERTENSION (HTN)

I. **BASIC PRINCIPLES**
   A. Increased blood pressure; may involve pulmonary (see chapter 9) or systemic circulation
   B. Systemic HTN is defined as pressure ≥ 140/90 mm Hg (normal ≤ 120/80 mm Hg); divided into primary or secondary types based on etiology

II. **PRIMARY HTN**
   A. HTN of unknown etiology (95% of cases)
   B. Risk factors include age, race (increased risk in African Americans, decreased risk in Asians), obesity, stress, lack of physical activity, and high-salt diet.

III. **SECONDARY HTN**
   A. HTN due to an identifiable etiology (5% of cases)
   B. Renal artery stenosis is a common cause (renovascular hypertension).
      1. Stenosis decreases blood flow to glomerulus.
      2. Juxtaglomerular apparatus (JGA) responds by secreting renin, which converts angiotensinogen to angiotensin I.
      3. Angiotensin I is converted to angiotensin II (ATII) by angiotensin converting enzyme (ACE).
      4. ATII raises blood pressure by (1) contracting arteriolar smooth muscle, increasing total peripheral resistance and (2) promoting adrenal release of aldosterone, which increases resorption of sodium in the distal convoluted tubule (expanding plasma volume).
      5. Leads to HTN with increased plasma renin and unilateral atrophy (due to low blood flow) of the affected kidney; neither feature is seen in primary hypertension.
   C. Important causes of stenosis include atherosclerosis (elderly males) and fibromuscular dysplasia (young females).

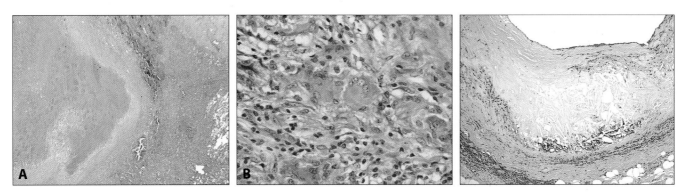

Fig. 7.4 Wegener granulomatosis. A, Necrotizing granuloma. B, Giant cells at edge of granuloma.   **Fig. 7.5** Atherosclerosis.

1. Fibromuscular dysplasia is a developmental defect of the blood vessel wall, resulting in irregular thickening of large- and medium-sized arteries, especially the renal artery.

IV. BENIGN AND MALIGNANT HTN

A. HTN can also be classified as benign or malignant.

B. Benign HTN is a mild or moderate elevation in blood pressure; most cases of HTN are benign.

    1. Clinically silent; vessels and organs are damaged slowly over time.

C. Malignant HTN is severe elevation in blood pressure (> 200/120 mm Hg); comprises < 5% of cases

    1. May arise from preexisting benign HTN or de novo

    2. Presents with acute end-organ damage (e.g., acute renal failure, headache, and papilledema) and is a medical emergency

ARTERIOSCLEROSIS

I. BASIC PRINCIPLES

A. Literally, "hard arteries;" due to thickening of the blood vessel wall

B. Three pathologic patterns—atherosclerosis, arteriolosclerosis, and Mönckeberg medial calcific sclerosis

II. ATHEROSCLEROSIS

A. Intimal plaque that obstructs blood flow

    1. Consists of a necrotic lipid core (mostly cholesterol) with a fibromuscular cap (Fig. 7.5); often undergoes dystrophic calcification

B. Involves large- and medium-sized arteries; abdominal aorta, coronary artery, popliteal artery, and internal carotid artery are commonly affected.

C. Risk factors for atherosclerosis are divided into modifiable and nonmodifiable.

    1. Modifiable risk factors include hypertension, hypercholesterolemia (LDL increases risk; HDL decreases risk), smoking, and diabetes.

    2. Nonmodifiable risk factors include age (number and severity of lesions increase with age), gender (increased risk in males and postmenopausal females; estrogen is protective), and genetics (multifactorial, but family history is highly predictive of risk).

D. Pathogenesis

    1. Damage to endothelium allows lipids to leak into the intima.

    2. Lipids are oxidized and then consumed by macrophages via scavenger receptors, resulting in foam cells.

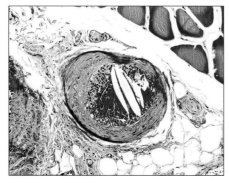

Fig. 7.6 Atherosclerotic embolus. (Courtesy of Professor A. Garfia)

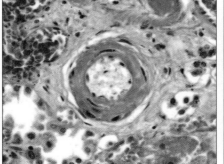

Fig. 7.7 Hyaline arteriolosclerosis.

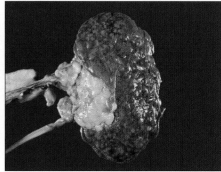

Fig. 7.8 Arteriolonephrosclerosis. (Courtesy of Jerome Taxy, MD)

3. Inflammation and healing leads to deposition of extracellular matrix and proliferation of smooth muscle.

E. Morphologic stages

1. Begins as fatty streaks (flat yellow lesions of the intima consisting of lipid-laden macrophages); arise early in life (present in most teenagers)
2. Progresses to atherosclerotic plaque

F. Complications of atherosclerosis account for > 50% of disease in Western countries.

1. Stenosis of medium-sized vessels results in impaired blood flow and ischemia leading to
   i. Peripheral vascular disease (lower extremity arteries, e.g., popliteal)
   ii. Angina (coronary arteries)
   iii. Ischemic bowel disease (mesenteric arteries)
2. Plaque rupture with thrombosis results in myocardial infarction (coronary arteries) and stroke (e.g., middle cerebral artery).
3. Plaque rupture with embolization results in atherosclerotic emboli, characterized by cholesterol crystals within the embolus (Fig. 7.6).
4. Weakening of vessel wall results in aneurysm (e.g., abdominal aorta).

III. ARTERIOLOSCLEROSIS

A. Narrowing of small arterioles; divided into hyaline and hyperplastic types

B. Hyaline arteriolosclerosis is caused by proteins leaking into the vessel wall, producing vascular thickening; proteins are seen as pink hyaline on microscopy (Fig. 7.7).

1. Consequence of long-standing benign hypertension or diabetes
2. Results in reduced vessel caliber with end-organ ischemia; classically produces glomerular scarring (arteriolonephrosclerosis, Fig. 7.8) that slowly progresses to chronic renal failure

C. Hyperplastic arteriolosclerosis involves thickening of vessel wall by hyperplasia of smooth muscle ('onion-skin' appearance, Fig. 7.9).

1. Consequence of malignant hypertension
2. Results in reduced vessel caliber with end-organ ischemia
3. May lead to fibrinoid necrosis of the vessel wall with hemorrhage; classically causes acute renal failure with a characteristic 'flea-bitten' appearance

IV. MÖNCKEBERG MEDIAL CALCIFIC SCLEROSIS

A. Calcification of the media of muscular (medium-sized) arteries; nonobstructive (Fig. 7.10A)

B. Not clinically significant; seen as an incidental finding on x-ray or mammography (Fig. 7.10B)

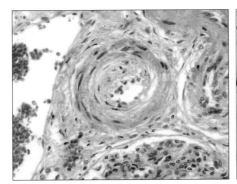

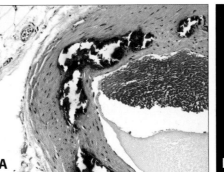

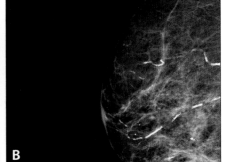

Fig. 7.9 Hyperplastic arteriolosclerosis.   **Fig. 7.10** Mönckeberg medial calcific sclerosis. **A**, Microscopic appearance. **B**, Mammogram.

AORTIC DISSECTION AND ANEURYSM

I. **AORTIC DISSECTION**
   A. Intimal tear with dissection of blood through media of the aortic wall (Fig. 7.11)
   B. Occurs in the proximal 10 cm of the aorta (high stress region) with preexisting weakness of the media
   C. Most common cause is hypertension (older adults); also associated with inherited defects of connective tissue (younger individuals)
      1. Hypertension results in hyaline arteriosclerosis of the vasa vasorum; decreased flow causes atrophy of the media.
      2. Marfan syndrome and Ehlers-Danlos syndrome classically lead to weakness of the connective tissue in the media (cystic medial necrosis).
   D. Presents as sharp, tearing chest pain that radiates to the back
   E. Complications include pericardial tamponade (most common cause of death), rupture with fatal hemorrhage, and obstruction of branching arteries (e.g., coronary or renal) with resultant end-organ ischemia.

II. **THORACIC ANEURYSM**
   A. Balloon-like dilation of the thoracic aorta
   B. Due to weakness in the aortic wall. Classically seen in tertiary syphilis; endarteritis of the vasa vasorum results in luminal narrowing, decreased flow, and atrophy of the vessel wall. Results in a 'tree-bark' appearance of the aorta (Fig. 7.12)
   C. Major complication is dilation of the aortic valve root, resulting in aortic valve insufficiency.
      1. Other complications include compression of mediastinal structures (e.g., airway or esophagus) and thrombosis/embolism.

III. **ABDOMINAL AORTIC ANEURYSM**
   A. Balloon-like dilation of the abdominal aorta; usually arises below the renal arteries, but above the aortic bifurcation (Fig. 7.13)
   B. Primarily due to atherosclerosis; classically seen in male smokers > 60 years old with hypertension
      1. Atherosclerosis increases the diffusion barrier to the media, resulting in atrophy and weakness of the vessel wall.
   C. Presents as a pulsatile abdominal mass that grows with time
   D. Major complication is rupture, especially when > 5 cm in diameter; presents with triad of hypotension, pulsatile abdominal mass, and flank pain
      1. Other complications include compression of local structures (e.g., ureter) and thrombosis/embolism.

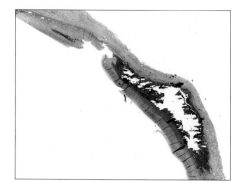

Fig. 7.11 Aortic dissection. (Courtesy of humpath. com)

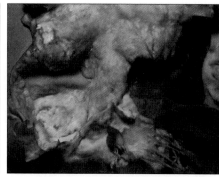

Fig. 7.12 'Tree-bark' appearance of aorta, due to syphilis. (Courtesy of Aliya Husain, MD)

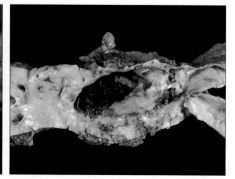

Fig, 7.13 Abdominal aortic aneurysm. (Courtesy of Aliya Husain, MD)

VASCULAR TUMORS

I. **HEMANGIOMA**
   A. Benign tumor comprised of blood vessels (Fig. 7.14)
   B. Commonly present at birth; often regresses during childhood
   C. Most often involves skin and liver

II. **ANGIOSARCOMA**
   A. Malignant proliferation of endothelial cells; highly aggressive
   B. Common sites include skin, breast, and liver.
      1. Liver angiosarcoma is associated with exposure to polyvinyl chloride, arsenic, and Thorotrast.

III. **KAPOSI SARCOMA**
   A. Low-grade malignant proliferation of endothelial cells; associated with HHV-8
   B. Presents as purple patches, plaques, and nodules on the skin (Fig. 7.15); may also involve visceral organs
   C. Classically seen in
      1. Older Eastern European males—tumor remains localized to skin; treatment involves surgical removal.
      2. AIDS—tumor spreads early; treatment is antiretroviral agents (to boost immune system).
      3. Transplant recipients—tumor spreads early; treatment involves decreasing immunosuppression.

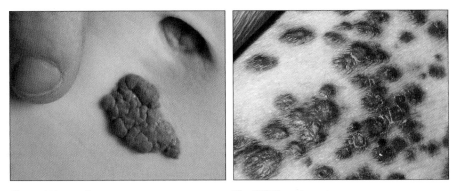

Fig. 7.14 Hemangioma.   **Fig. 7.15** Kaposi sarcoma.

Cardiac Pathology

8

ISCHEMIC HEART DISEASE (IHD)

I. **BASIC PRINCIPLES**

  A. Group of syndromes related to myocardial ischemia; IHD is the leading cause of death in the US.

  B. Usually due to atherosclerosis of coronary arteries, which decreases blood flow to the myocardium

    1. Risk factors for IHD are similar to those of atherosclerosis; incidence increases with age.

II. **ANGINA**

  A. Stable angina is chest pain that arises with exertion or emotional stress.

    1. Due to atherosclerosis of coronary arteries with > 70% stenosis; decreased blood flow is not able to meet the metabolic demands of the myocardium during exertion.

    2. Represents reversible injury to myocytes (no necrosis)

    3. Presents as chest pain (lasting < 20 minutes) that radiates to the left arm or jaw, diaphoresis, and shortness of breath

    4. EKG shows ST-segment depression due to subendocardial ischemia.

    5. Relieved by rest or nitroglycerin

  B. Unstable angina is chest pain that occurs at rest.

    1. Usually due to rupture of an atherosclerotic plaque with thrombosis and *incomplete* occlusion of a coronary artery (Fig. 8.1A).

    2. Represents reversible injury to myocytes (no necrosis)

    3. EKG shows ST-segment depression due to subendocardial ischemia.

    4. Relieved by nitroglycerin

    5. High risk of progression to myocardial infarction

  C. Prinzmetal angina is episodic chest pain unrelated to exertion.

    1. Due to coronary artery vasospasm

    2. Represents reversible injury to myocytes (no necrosis)

    3. EKG shows ST-segment elevation due to transmural ischemia.

    4. Relieved by nitroglycerin or calcium channel blockers

III. **MYOCARDIAL INFARCTION**

  A. Necrosis of cardiac myocytes

  B. Usually due to rupture of an atherosclerotic plaque with thrombosis and *complete* occlusion of a coronary artery (Fig. 8.1B)

    1. Other causes include coronary artery vasospasm (due to Prinzmetal angina or cocaine use), emboli, and vasculitis (e.g., Kawasaki disease).

  C. Clinical features include severe, crushing chest pain (lasting > 20 minutes) that radiates to the left arm or jaw, diaphoresis, and dyspnea; symptoms are not relieved by nitroglycerin.

  D. Infarction usually involves the left ventricle (LV); right ventricle (RV) and both atria are generally spared.

1. Occlusion of left anterior descending artery (LAD) leads to infarction of the anterior wall and anterior septum of the LV; LAD is the most commonly involved artery in MI (45% of cases).
2. Occlusion of right coronary artery (RCA) leads to infarction of the posterior wall, posterior septum, and papillary muscles of the LV; RCA is the 2nd most commonly involved artery in MI.
3. Occlusion of left circumflex artery leads to infarction of lateral wall of the LV.

E. Initial phase of infarction leads to subendocardial necrosis involving < 50% of the myocardial thickness (subendocardial infarction, Fig. 8.2); EKG shows ST-segment depression.
   1. Continued or severe ischemia leads to transmural necrosis involving most of the myocardial wall (transmural infarction); EKG shows ST-segment elevation.

F. Laboratory tests detect elevated cardiac enzymes.
   1. Troponin I is the most sensitive and specific marker (gold standard) for MI. Levels rise 2–4 hours after infarction, peak at 24 hours, and return to normal by 7–10 days.
   2. CK-MB is useful for detecting reinfarction that occurs days after an initial MI; creatine kinase MB (CK-MB) levels rise 4–6 hours after infarction, peak at 24 hours, and return to normal by 72 hours.

G. Treatment includes
   1. Aspirin and/or heparin—limits thrombosis
   2. Supplemental O_2—minimizes ischemia
   3. Nitrates—vasodilate veins and coronary arteries
   4. β-blocker—slows heart rate, decreasing O_2 demand and risk for arrhythmia
   5. ACE inhibitor—decreases LV dilation
   6. Fibrinolysis or angioplasty—opens blocked vessel
      i. Reperfusion of irreversibly-damaged cells results in calcium influx, leading to hypercontraction of myofibrils (contraction band necrosis, Fig. 8.3).
      ii. Return of oxygen and inflammatory cells may lead to free radical generation, further damaging myocytes (reperfusion injury).

H. Complications of myocardial infarction are closely related to gross and microscopic changes (Table 8.1).

Table 8.1: Morphologic Changes in Myocardial Infarction

TIME FROM INFARCTION	GROSS CHANGES	MICROSCOPIC CHANGES	COMPLICATIONS
< 4 hours	None	None	Cardiogenic shock (massive infarction), congestive heart failure, and arrhythmia
4–24 hours	Dark discoloration	Coagulative necrosis (Fig. 8.4A)	Arrhythmia
1–3 days	Yellow pallor	Neutrophils (Fig. 8.4B)	Fibrinous pericarditis (Fig. 8.5A); presents as chest pain with friction rub
4–7 days	Yellow pallor	Macrophages	Rupture of ventricular free wall (Fig. 8.5B; leads to cardiac tamponade), interventricular septum (leads to shunt), or papillary muscle (Fig. 8.5C; leads to mitral insufficiency)
1–3 weeks	Red border emerges as granulation tissue enters from edge of infarct.	Granulation tissue with plump fibroblasts, collagen, and blood vessels	
Months	White scar (Fig. 8.6A)	Fibrosis (Fig. 8.6B)	Aneurysm (Fig. 8.7), mural thrombus, or Dressler syndrome

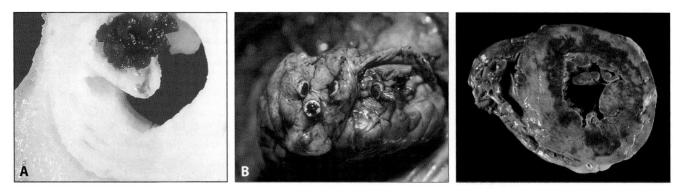

Fig. 8.1 Thrombosis of coronary artery. **A**, Incomplete occlusion. **B**, Complete occlusion. (Courtesy of Aliya Husain, MD)

Fig. 8.2 Early infarction (< 1 day old), predominantly subendocardial. (Courtesy of Jerome Taxy, MD)

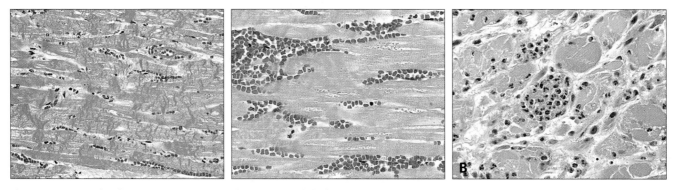

Fig. 8.3 Contraction band necrosis.

Fig. 8.4 Myocardial infarction. **A**, Coagulative necrosis of myocardium. **B**, Neutrophilic infiltrate.

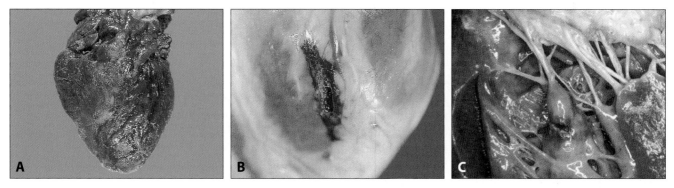

Fig. 8.5 Complications of myocardial infarction. **A**, Fibrinous pericarditis. **B**, Rupture of ventricular free wall. **C**, Rupture of papillary muscle. (Courtesy of Aliya Husain, MD)

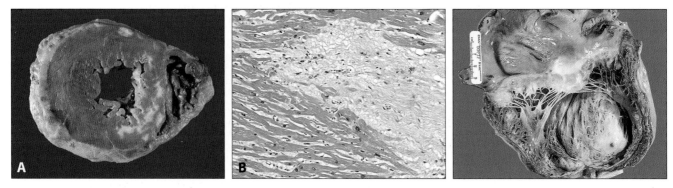

Fig. 8.6 Myocardial scar. **A**, Gross appearance. **B**, Microscopic appearance. (A, Courtesy of Ajit Paintal, MD)

Fig. 8.7 Ventricular aneurysm.

IV. **SUDDEN CARDIAC DEATH**
  A. Unexpected death due to cardiac disease; occurs without symptoms or < 1 hour after symptoms arise
    1. Usually due to fatal ventricular arrhythmia
  B. Most common etiology is acute ischemia; 90% of patients have preexisting severe atherosclerosis.
    1. Less common causes include mitral valve prolapse, cardiomyopathy, and cocaine abuse.

V. **CHRONIC ISCHEMIC HEART DISEASE**
  A. Poor myocardial function due to chronic ischemic damage (with or without infarction); progresses to congestive heart failure (CHF)

CONGESTIVE HEART FAILURE (CHF)

I. **BASIC PRINCIPLES**
  A. Pump failure; divided into right- and left-sided failure

II. **LEFT-SIDED HEART FAILURE**
  A. Causes include ischemia, hypertension, dilated cardiomyopathy, myocardial infarction, and restrictive cardiomyopathy.
  B. Clinical features are due to decreased forward perfusion and pulmonary congestion.
    1. Pulmonary congestion leads to pulmonary edema.
      i. Results in dyspnea, paroxysmal nocturnal dyspnea (due to increased venous return when lying flat), orthopnea, and crackles
      ii. Small, congested capillaries may burst, leading to intraalveolar hemorrhage; marked by hemosiderin-laden macrophages ('heart-failure' cells, Fig. 8.8)
    2. Decreased flow to kidneys leads to activation of renin-angiotensin system.
      i. Fluid retention exacerbates CHF.
  C. Mainstay of treatment is ACE inhibitor.

III. **RIGHT-SIDED HEART FAILURE**
  A. Most commonly due to left-sided heart failure; other important causes include left-to-right shunt and chronic lung disease (cor pulmonale).
  B. Clinical features are due to congestion.
    1. Jugular venous distension
    2. Painful hepatosplenomegaly with characteristic 'nutmeg' liver (Fig. 8.9); may lead to cardiac cirrhosis
    3. Dependent pitting edema (due to increased hydrostatic pressure)

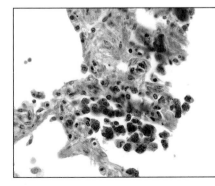

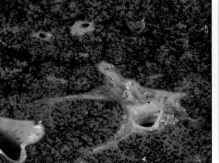

Fig. 8.8 Hemosiderin-laden macrophages ('heart failure' cells).   **Fig. 8.9** 'Nutmeg' liver, congestive heart failure.   **Fig. 8.10** 'Boot-shaped' heart, tetralogy of Fallot.

CONGENITAL DEFECTS

I. **BASIC PRINCIPLES**
   A. Arise during embryogenesis (usually weeks 3 through 8); seen in 1% of live births
      1. Most defects are sporadic.
   B. Often result in shunting between left (systemic) and right (pulmonary) circulations.
   C. Defects with left-to-right shunting may be relatively asymptomatic at birth, but the shunt can eventually reverse.
      1. Increased flow through the pulmonary circulation results in hypertrophy of pulmonary vessels and pulmonary hypertension.
      2. Increased pulmonary resistance eventually results in reversal of shunt, leading to late cyanosis (Eisenmenger syndrome) with right ventricular hypertrophy, polycythemia, and clubbing.
   D. Defects with right-to-left shunting usually present as cyanosis shortly after birth.

II. **VENTRICULAR SEPTAL DEFECT (VSD)**
   A. Defect in the septum that divides the right and left ventricles
      1. Most common congenital heart defect
      2. Associated with fetal alcohol syndrome
   B. Results in left-to-right shunt; size of defect determines extent of shunting and age at presentation. Small defects are often asymptomatic; large defects can lead to Eisenmenger syndrome.
   C. Treatment involves surgical closure; small defects may close spontaneously.

III. **ATRIAL SEPTAL DEFECT (ASD)**
   A. Defect in the septum that divides right and left atria; most common type is ostium secundum (90% of cases).
   B. Ostium primum type is associated with Down syndrome.
   C. Results in left-to-right shunt and split S_2 on auscultation (increased blood in right heart delays closure of pulmonary valve)
   D. Paradoxical emboli are an important complication.

IV. **PATENT DUCTUS ARTERIOSUS (PDA)**
   A. Failure of ductus arteriosus to close; associated with congenital rubella
   B. Results in left-to-right shunt between the aorta and the pulmonary artery
      1. During development, the ductus arteriosus normally shunts blood from the pulmonary artery to the aorta, bypassing the lungs.
   C. Asymptomatic at birth with continuous 'machine-like' murmur; may lead to Eisenmenger syndrome, resulting in lower extremity cyanosis
   D. Treatment involves indomethacin, which decreases PGE, resulting in PDA closure (PGE maintains patency of the ductus arteriosus).

V. **TETRALOGY OF FALLOT**
   A. Characterized by (1) stenosis of the right ventricular outflow tract, (2) right ventricular hypertrophy, (3) VSD, and (4) an aorta that overrides the VSD
   B. Right-to-left shunt leads to early cyanosis; degree of stenosis determines the extent of shunting and cyanosis.
   C. Patients learn to squat in response to a cyanotic spell; increased arterial resistance decreases shunting and allows more blood to reach the lungs.
   D. 'Boot-shaped' heart on x-ray (Fig. 8.10)

VI. **TRANSPOSITION OF THE GREAT VESSELS**
   A. Characterized by pulmonary artery arising from the left ventricle and aorta arising from the right ventricle

    B. Associated with maternal diabetes

    C. Presents with early cyanosis; pulmonary and systemic circuits do not mix.

        1. Creation of shunt (allowing blood to mix) after birth is required for survival.

        2. PGE can be administered to maintain a PDA until definitive surgical repair is performed.

    D. Results in hypertrophy of the right ventricle and atrophy of the left ventricle

VII. TRUNCUS ARTERIOSUS

    A. Characterized by a single large vessel arising from both ventricles

        1. Truncus fails to divide.

    B. Presents with early cyanosis; deoxygenated blood from right ventricle mixes with oxygenated blood from left ventricle before pulmonary and aortic circulations separate.

VIII. TRICUSPID ATRESIA

    A. Tricuspid valve orifice fails to develop; right ventricle is hypoplastic.

    B. Often associated with ASD, resulting in a right-to-left shunt; presents with early cyanosis.

IX. COARCTATION OF THE AORTA

    A. Narrowing of the aorta (Fig. 8.11A); classically divided into infantile and adult forms

    B. Infantile form is associated with a PDA; coarctation lies after (distal to) the aortic arch, but before (proximal to) the PDA.

        1. Presents as lower extremity cyanosis in infants, often at birth

        2. Associated with Turner syndrome

    C. Adult form is not associated with a PDA; coarctation lies after (distal to) the aortic arch.

        1. Presents as hypertension in the upper extremities and hypotension with weak pulses in the lower extremities; classically discovered in adulthood

        2. Collateral circulation develops across the intercostal arteries; engorged arteries cause 'notching' of ribs on x-ray (Fig. 8.11B).

        3. Associated with bicuspid aortic valve

VALVULAR DISORDERS

I. BASIC PRINCIPLES

    A. The heart has four valves (tricuspid, pulmonary, mitral, and aortic) that prevent backflow.

    B. Valvular lesions generally result in stenosis (decreased caliber of the valve orifice) or regurgitation (backflow).

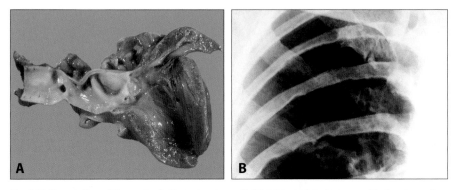

Fig. 8.11 Coarctation of the aorta. **A,** Gross specimen. **B,** 'Notching of ribs' on x-ray. (A, Courtesy of Aliya Husain, MD. B, Courtesy of *Images Paediatr Cardiol* 2009;38:7–9)

II. ACUTE RHEUMATIC FEVER

A. Systemic complication of pharyngitis due to group A β-hemolytic streptococci; affects children 2–3 weeks after an episode of streptococcal pharyngitis ("strep throat")

B. Caused by molecular mimicry; bacterial M protein resembles proteins in human tissue.

C. Diagnosis is based on Jones criteria.

1. Evidence of prior group A β-hemolytic streptococcal infection (e.g., elevated ASO or anti-DNase B titers) with the presence of major and minor criteria

2. Minor criteria are nonspecific and include fever and elevated ESR.

3. Major criteria

   i. Migratory polyarthritis—swelling and pain in a large joint (e.g., wrist, knees, ankles) that resolves within days and "migrates" to involve another large joint

   ii. Pancarditis

      a. Endocarditis—Mitral valve is involved more commonly than the aortic valve. Characterized by small vegetations along lines of closure that lead to regurgitation (Fig. 8.12A)

      b. Myocarditis with Aschoff bodies that are characterized by foci of chronic inflammation, reactive histiocytes with slender, wavy nuclei (Anitschkow cells), giant cells, and fibrinoid material (Fig. 8.12B,C); myocarditis is the most common cause of death during the acute phase.

      c. Pericarditis—leads to friction rub and chest pain

   iii. Subcutaneous nodules

   iv. Erythema marginatum—annular, nonpruritic rash with erythematous borders, commonly involving trunk and limbs

   v. Sydenham chorea (rapid, involuntary muscle movements)

D. Acute attack usually resolves, but may progress to chronic rheumatic heart disease; repeat exposure to group A β-hemolytic streptococci results in relapse of the acute phase and increases risk for chronic disease.

III. CHRONIC RHEUMATIC HEART DISEASE

A. Valve scarring that arises as a consequence of rheumatic fever

B. Results in stenosis with a classic 'fish-mouth' appearance

1. Almost always involves the mitral valve; leads to thickening of chordae tendineae and cusps

2. Occasionally involves the aortic valve; leads to fusion of the commissures (Fig. 8.13)

3. Other valves are less commonly involved.

C. Complications include infectious endocarditis.

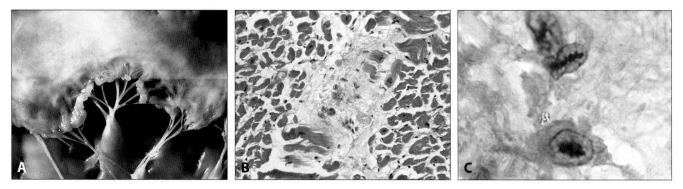

Fig. 8.12 Acute rheumatic heart disease. **A**, Mitral valve vegetations. **B**, Aschoff body involving myocardium. **C**, Anitschkow cells. (A, Courtesy of Aliya Husain, MD. B, Courtesy of Ed Uthman, MD)

IV. **AORTIC STENOSIS**
   A. Narrowing of the aortic valve orifice (Fig. 8.14)
   B. Usually due to fibrosis and calcification from "wear and tear"
      1. Presents in late adulthood (> 60 years)
      2. Bicuspid aortic valve increases risk and hastens disease onset. A normal aortic valve has three cusps; fewer cusps results in increased "wear and tear" on each cusp.
   C. May also arise as a consequence of chronic rheumatic valve disease; coexisting mitral stenosis and fusion of the aortic valve commissures distinguish rheumatic disease from "wear and tear."
   D. Cardiac compensation leads to a prolonged asymptomatic stage during which a systolic ejection click followed by a crescendo-decrescendo murmur is heard.
   E. Complications include
      1. Concentric left ventricular hypertrophy—may progress to cardiac failure
      2. Angina and syncope with exercise—Limited ability to increase blood flow across the stenotic valve leads to decreased perfusion of the myocardium and brain.
      3. Microangiopathic hemolytic anemia—RBCs are damaged (producing schistocytes) while crossing the calcified valve.
   F. Treatment is valve replacement after onset of complications.

V. **AORTIC REGURGITATION**
   A. Backflow of blood from the aorta into the left ventricle during diastole
   B. Arises due to aortic root dilation (e.g., syphilitic aneurysm and aortic dissection) or valve damage (e.g., infectious endocarditis); most common cause is isolated root dilation
   C. Clinical features include
      1. Early, blowing diastolic murmur
      2. Hyperdynamic circulation due to increased pulse pressure
         i. Pulse pressure is the difference between systolic and diastolic pressures.
         ii. Diastolic pressure decreases due to regurgitation, while systolic pressure increases due to increased stroke volume.
         iii. Presents with bounding pulse (water-hammer pulse), pulsating nail bed (Quincke pulse), and head bobbing
      3. Results in LV dilation and eccentric hypertrophy (due to volume overload)
   D. Treatment is valve replacement once LV dysfunction develops.

VI. **MITRAL VALVE PROLAPSE**
   A. Ballooning of mitral valve into left atrium during systole
      1. Seen in 2–3% of US adults

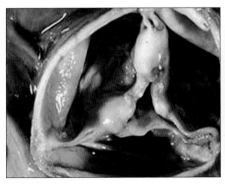

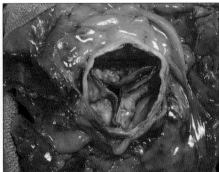

Fig. 8.13 Fusion of aortic valve commissures, chronic rheumatic heart disease. (Courtesy of Aliya Husain, MD)

Fig. 8.14 Aortic stenosis. (Courtesy of Aliya Husain, MD)

B. Due to myxoid degeneration (accumulation of ground substance) of the valve, making it floppy (Fig. 8.15)
   1. Etiology is unknown; may be seen in Marfan syndrome or Ehlers-Danlos syndrome
C. Presents with an incidental mid-systolic click followed by a regurgitation murmur; usually asymptomatic
   1. Click and murmur become softer with squatting (increased systemic resistance decreases left ventricular emptying).
D. Complications are rare, but include infectious endocarditis, arrhythmia, and severe mitral regurgitation.
E. Treatment is valve replacement.

VII. MITRAL REGURGITATION
A. Reflux of blood from the left ventricle into the left atrium during systole
B. Usually arises as a complication of mitral valve prolapse; other causes include LV dilatation (e.g., left-sided cardiac failure), infective endocarditis, acute rheumatic heart disease, and papillary muscle rupture after a myocardial infarction.
C. Clinical features
   1. Holosystolic "blowing" murmur; louder with squatting (increased systemic resistance decreases left ventricular emptying) and expiration (increased return to left atrium)
   2. Results in volume overload and left-sided heart failure

VIII. MITRAL STENOSIS
A. Narrowing of the mitral valve orifice
   1. Usually due to chronic rheumatic valve disease
B. Clinical features
   1. Opening snap followed by diastolic rumble
   2. Volume overload leads to dilatation of the left atrium, resulting in
      i. Pulmonary congestion with edema and alveolar hemorrhage
      ii. Pulmonary hypertension and eventual right-sided heart failure
      iii. Atrial fibrillation with associated risk for mural thrombi (Fig. 8.16)

ENDOCARDITIS

I. BASIC PRINCIPLES
A. Inflammation of endocardium that lines the surface of cardiac valves; usually due to bacterial infection
B. *Streptococcus viridans* is the most common overall cause. It is a low-virulence organism that infects previously damaged valves (e.g., chronic rheumatic heart

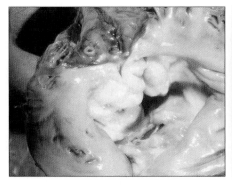

Fig. 8.15 Mitral valve prolapse. (Courtesy of Aliya Husain, MD)

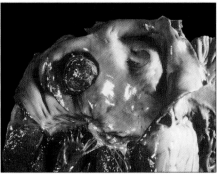

Fig. 8.16 Mural thrombus involving left atrium. (Courtesy of Aliya Husain, MD)

disease and mitral valve prolapse). Results in small vegetations that do not destroy the valve (subacute endocarditis)

1. Damaged endocardial surface develops thrombotic vegetations (platelets and fibrin).
2. Transient bacteremia leads to trapping of bacteria in the vegetations; prophylactic antibiotics decrease risk of endocarditis.

C. *Staphylococcus aureus* is the most common cause in IV drug abusers.
   1. High-virulence organism that infects normal valves, most commonly the tricuspid.
   2. Results in large vegetations that destroy the valve (acute endocarditis, Fig. 8.17)

D. *Staphylococcus epidermidis* is associated with endocarditis of prosthetic valves.

E. *Streptococcus bovis* is associated with endocarditis in patients with underlying colorectal carcinoma.

F. HACEK organisms (*Haemophilus, Actinobacillus, Cardiobacterium, Eikenella, Kingella*) are associated with endocarditis with negative blood cultures.

G. Clinical features of bacterial endocarditis include
   1. Fever—due to bacteremia
   2. Murmur—due to vegetations on heart valve
   3. Janeway lesions (erythematous nontender lesions on palms and soles), Osler nodes (tender lesions on fingers or toes), and splinter hemorrhages in nail bed—due to embolization of septic vegetations
   4. Anemia of chronic disease—due to chronic inflammation

H. Laboratory findings
   1. Positive blood cultures
   2. Anemia of chronic disease ($\downarrow$ Hb, $\downarrow$MCV; $\uparrow$ ferritin, $\downarrow$ TIBC, $\downarrow$ serum iron, and $\downarrow$ % saturation)
   3. Transesophageal echocardiogram is useful for detecting lesions on valves.

I. Nonbacterial thrombotic endocarditis is due to sterile vegetations that arise in association with a hypercoagulable state or underlying adenocarcinoma. Vegetations arise on the mitral valve along lines of closure and result in mitral regurgitation.

J. Libman-Sacks endocarditis is due to sterile vegetations that arise in association with SLE. Vegetations are present on the surface and undersurface of the mitral valve and result in mitral regurgitation.

CARDIOMYOPATHY

I. **BASIC PRINCIPLES**
   A. Group of myocardial diseases that result in cardiac dysfunction

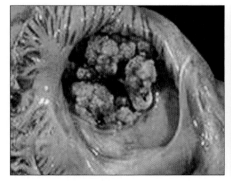

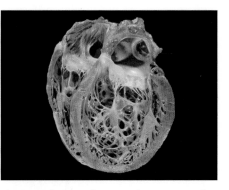

Fig. 8.17 Large vegetations involving tricuspid valve. (Courtesy of Aliya Husain, MD)

Fig. 8.18 Dilated cardiomyopathy. (Courtesy of Jamie Steinmetz, MD)

II. DILATED CARDIOMYOPATHY

A. Dilation of all four chambers of the heart (Fig. 8.18); most common form of cardiomyopathy

B. Results in systolic dysfunction (ventricles cannot pump), leading to biventricular CHF; complications include mitral and tricuspid valve regurgitation and arrhythmia.

C. Most commonly idiopathic; other causes include

1. Genetic mutation (usually autosomal dominant)
2. Myocarditis (usually due to coxsackie A or B)—characterized by a lymphocytic infiltrate in the myocardium (Fig. 8.19); results in chest pain, arrhythmia with sudden death, or heart failure. Dilated cardiomyopathy is a late complication.
3. Alcohol abuse
4. Drugs (e.g., doxorubicin)
5. Pregnancy—seen during late pregnancy or soon (weeks to months) after childbirth
6. Hemochromatosis

D. Treatment is heart transplant.

III. HYPERTROPHIC CARDIOMYOPATHY

A. Massive hypertrophy of the left ventricle

B. Usually due to genetic mutations in sarcomere proteins; most common form is autosomal dominant.

C. Clinical features include

1. Decreased cardiac output—Left ventricular hypertrophy leads to diastolic dysfunction (ventricle cannot fill).
2. Sudden death due to ventricular arrhythmias; hypertrophic cardiomyopathy is a common cause of sudden death in young athletes.
3. Syncope with exercise—Subaortic hypertrophy of the ventricular septum results in functional aortic stenosis.

D. Biopsy shows myofiber hypertrophy with disarray (Fig. 8.20).

IV. RESTRICTIVE CARDIOMYOPATHY

A. Decreased compliance of the ventricular endomyocardium that restricts filling during diastole

B. Causes include amyloidosis, sarcoidosis, endocardial fibroelastosis (children, Fig. 8.21), and Loeffler syndrome (endomyocardial fibrosis with an eosinophilic infiltrate and eosinophilia).

C. Presents as congestive heart failure; classic finding is low-voltage EKG with diminished QRS amplitude.

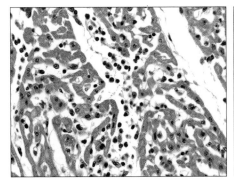

Fig. 8.19 Myocarditis.

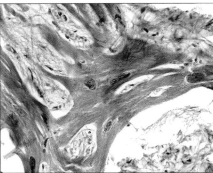

Fig. 8.20 Myofiber disarray, hypertrophic cardiomyopathy.

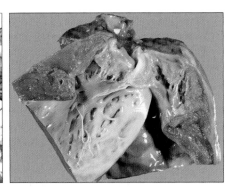

Fig. 8.21 Endocardial fibroelastosis. (Courtesy of humpath.com)

CARDIAC TUMORS

I. **MYXOMA**
   A. Benign mesenchymal tumor with a gelatinous appearance and abundant ground substance on histology
      1. Most common primary cardiac tumor in adults
   B. Usually forms a pedunculated mass in the left atrium that causes syncope due to obstruction of the mitral valve

II. **RHABDOMYOMA**
   A. Benign hamartoma of cardiac muscle
      1. Most common primary cardiac tumor in children; associated with tuberous sclerosis
   B. Usually arises in the ventricle

III. **METASTASIS**
   A. Metastatic tumors are more common in the heart than primary tumors.
      1. Common metastases to the heart include breast and lung carcinoma, melanoma, and lymphoma.
   B. Most commonly involve the pericardium, resulting in a pericardial effusion

9

Respiratory Tract Pathology

NASOPHARYNX

I. **RHINITIS**
   A. Inflammation of the nasal mucosa; rhinovirus is the most common cause.
   B. Presents with sneezing, congestion, and runny nose (common cold)
   C. Allergic rhinitis is a subtype of rhinitis due to a type I hypersensitivity reaction (e.g., to pollen)
      1. Characterized by an inflammatory infiltrate with eosinophils
      2. Associated with asthma and eczema

II. **NASAL POLYP**
   A. Protrusion of edematous, inflamed nasal mucosa
   B. Usually secondary to repeated bouts of rhinitis; also occurs in cystic fibrosis and aspirin-intolerant asthma
      1. Aspirin-intolerant asthma is characterized by the triad of asthma, aspirin-induced bronchospasms, and nasal polyps; seen in 10% of asthmatic adults

III. **ANGIOFIBROMA**
   A. Benign tumor of nasal mucosa composed of large blood vessels and fibrous tissue; classically seen in adolescent males
   B. Presents with profuse epistaxis

IV. **NASOPHARYNGEAL CARCINOMA**
   A. Malignant tumor of nasopharyngeal epithelium
   B. Associated with EBV; classically seen in African children and Chinese adults
   C. Biopsy usually reveals pleomorphic keratin-positive epithelial cells (poorly differentiated squamous cell carcinoma) in a background of lymphocytes.
   D. Often presents with involvement of cervical lymph nodes

LARYNX

I. **ACUTE EPIGLOTTITIS**
   A. Inflammation of the epiglottis (Fig. 9.1); *H influenzae* type b is the most common cause, especially in nonimmunized children.
   B. Presents with high fever, sore throat, drooling with dysphagia, muffled voice, and inspiratory stridor; risk of airway obstruction

II. **LARYNGOTRACHEOBRONCHITIS (CROUP)**
   A. Inflammation of the upper airway; parainfluenza virus is the most common cause.
   B. Presents with a hoarse, "barking" cough and inspiratory stridor

III. **VOCAL CORD NODULE (SINGER'S NODULE)**
   A. Nodule that arises on the true vocal cord
   B. Due to excessive use of vocal cords; usually bilateral (Fig. 9.2A)
      1. Composed of degenerative (myxoid) connective tissue (Fig. 9.2B)

C. Presents with hoarseness; resolves with resting of voice

IV. LARYNGEAL PAPILLOMA
A. Benign papillary tumor of the vocal cord
B. Due to HPV 6 and 11; papillomas are usually single in adults and multiple in children.
C. Presents with hoarseness

V. LARYNGEAL CARCINOMA
A. Squamous cell carcinoma usually arising from the epithelial lining of the vocal cord
B. Risk factors are alcohol and tobacco; can rarely arise from a laryngeal papilloma
C. Presents with hoarseness; other signs include cough and stridor.

Pain
Bradykinin
Prostaglandin E₂

PULMONARY INFECTIONS

I. PNEUMONIA
A. Infection of the lung parenchyma
B. Occurs when normal defenses are impaired (e.g., impaired cough reflex, damage to mucociliary escalator, or mucus plugging)
C. Clinical features include fever and chills, productive cough with yellow-green (pus) or rusty (bloody) sputum, tachypnea with pleuritic chest pain, decreased breath sounds, dullness to percussion, and elevated WBC count. *when you breath in you stretch pleura - pain*
D. Diagnosis is made by chest x-ray, sputum gram stain and culture, and blood cultures.
E. Three patterns are classically seen on chest x-ray: lobar pneumonia, bronchopneumonia, and interstitial pneumonia.

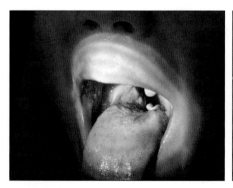

Fig. 9.1 Acute epiglottitis. (Courtesy of Stephanie Rozell, MD)

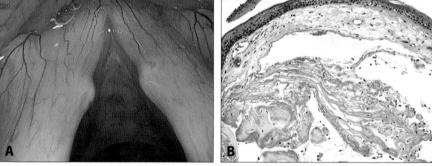

Fig. 9.2 Vocal cord nodules. **A**, Gross appearance. **B**, Microscopic appearance. (B, Reproduced from wikipedia.org, CCBY-SA 3.0)

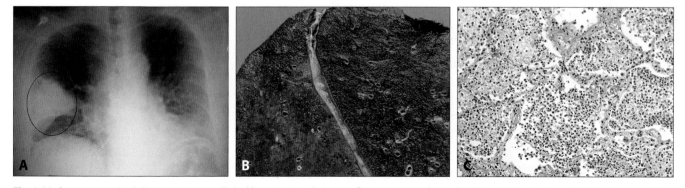

Fig. 9.3 Lobar pneumonia. **A**, X-ray appearance. **B**, Red hepatization. **C**, Acute inflammation involving alveolar sacs. (A, Courtesy of James Heilman, MD, Wikipedia. B, Courtesy of Yale Rosen, MD)

II. **LOBAR PNEUMONIA**
   A. Characterized by consolidation of an entire lobe of the lung (Fig. 9.3A)
   B. Usually bacterial; most common causes are *Streptococcus pneumoniae* (95%) and *Klebsiella pneumoniae* (Table 9.1)
   C. Classic gross phases of lobar pneumonia
      1. Congestion—due to congested vessels and edema
      2. Red hepatization—due to exudate, neutrophils, and hemorrhage filling the alveolar air spaces, giving the normally spongy lung a solid consistency (Fig. 9.3B,C)
      3. Gray hepatization—due to degradation of red cells within the exudate
      4. Resolution
         ⌐↝Type II pneumocytes

III. **BRONCHOPNEUMONIA**
   A. Characterized by scattered patchy consolidation centered around bronchioles; often multifocal and bilateral (Fig. 9.4)
   B. Caused by a variety of bacterial organisms (Table 9.2)

IV. **INTERSTITIAL (ATYPICAL) PNEUMONIA** = connective tissue of lungs / alveoli
   A. Characterized by diffuse interstitial infiltrates (Fig. 9.5)
   B. Presents with relatively mild upper respiratory symptoms (minimal sputum and low fever); 'atypical' presentation
   C. Caused by bacteria or viruses (Table 9.3)

V. **ASPIRATION PNEUMONIA**
   A. Seen in patients at risk for aspiration (e.g., alcoholics and comatose patients)
   B. Most often due to anaerobic bacteria in the oropharynx (e.g., *Bacteroides*, *Fusobacterium*, and *Peptococcus*)

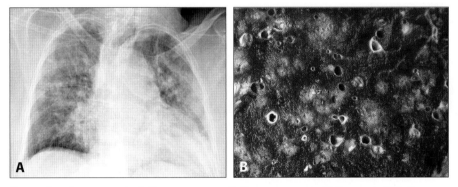

Fig. 9.4 Bronchopneumonia. **A**, X-ray appearance. **B**, Gross appearance. (B, Courtesy of Yale Rosen, MD)

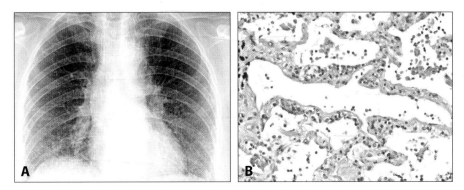

Fig. 9.5 Interstitial pneumonia. **A**, X-ray appearance. **B**, Inflammatory infiltrate involving interstitium.

Table 9.1: Causes of Lobar Pneumonia

ORGANISM	HIGH-YIELD ASSOCIATIONS
Streptococcus pneumoniae	Most common cause of community-acquired pneumonia and secondary pneumonia (bacterial pneumonia superimposed on a viral upper respiratory tract infection); usually seen in middle-aged adults and elderly
Klebsiella pneumoniae	Enteric flora that is aspirated; affects malnourished and debilitated individuals, especially elderly in nursing homes, alcoholics, and diabetics. Thick mucoid capsule results in gelatinous sputum (currant jelly); often complicated by abscess

Table 9.2: Causes of Bronchopneumonia

ORGANISM	HIGH-YIELD ASSOCIATIONS
Staphylococcus aureus	2nd most common cause of secondary pneumonia; often complicated by abscess or empyema = pus in pleural space
Haemophilus influenzae	Common cause of secondary pneumonia and pneumonia superimposed on COPD (leads to exacerbation of COPD)
Pseudomonas aeruginosa	Pneumonia in cystic fibrosis patients
Moraxella catarrhalis	Community-acquired pneumonia and pneumonia superimposed on COPD (leads to exacerbation of COPD)
Legionella pneumophila	Community-acquired pneumonia, pneumonia superimposed on COPD, or pneumonia in immunocompromised states; transmitted from water source Intracellular organism that is best visualized by silver stain

Table 9.3: Causes of Interstitial (Atypical) Pneumonia

ORGANISM	HIGH-YIELD ASSOCIATIONS
Mycoplasma pneumoniae	Most common cause of atypical pneumonia, usually affects young adults (classically, military recruits or college students living in a dormitory). Complications include autoimmune hemolytic anemia (IgM against I antigen on RBCs causes cold hemolytic anemia) and erythema multiforme. Not visible on gram stain due to lack of cell wall
Chlamydia pneumoniae	Second most common cause of atypical pneumonia in young adults
Respiratory syncytial virus (RSV)	Most common cause of atypical pneumonia in infants
Cytomegalovirus (CMV)	Atypical pneumonia with posttransplant immunosuppressive therapy
Influenza virus	Atypical pneumonia in the elderly, immunocompromised, and those with preexisting lung disease. Also increases the risk for superimposed *S aureus or H influenzae* bacterial pneumonia
Coxiella burnetii	Atypical pneumonia with high fever (Q fever); seen in farmers and veterinarians (*Coxiella* spores are deposited on cattle by ticks or are present in cattle placentas). *Coxiella* is a rickettsial organism, but it is distinct from most rickettsiae because it (1) causes pneumonia, (2) does not require arthropod vector for transmission (survives as highly heat-resistant endospores), and (3) does not produce a skin rash.

C. Classically results in a right lower lobe abscess
    1. Anatomically, the right main stem bronchus branches at a less acute angle than the left.

VI. TUBERCULOSIS (TB)
A. Due to inhalation of aerosolized *Mycobacterium tuberculosis*
B. Primary TB arises with initial exposure.
    1. Results in focal, caseating necrosis in the lower lobe of the lung and hilar lymph nodes that undergoes fibrosis and calcification, forming a Ghon complex (Fig. 9.6A)
    2. Primary TB is generally asymptomatic, but leads to a positive PPD.
C. Secondary TB arises with reactivation of *Mycobacterium tuberculosis*.
    1. Reactivation is commonly due to AIDS; may also be seen with aging
    2. Occurs at apex of lung (relatively poor lymphatic drainage and high oxygen tension)
    3. Forms cavitary foci of caseous necrosis; may also lead to miliary pulmonary TB or tuberculous bronchopneumonia   *↳ scattered over lung*
    4. Clinical features include fevers and night sweats, cough with hemoptysis, and weight loss.
    5. Biopsy reveals caseating granulomas; AFB stain reveals acid-fast bacilli (Fig. 9.6B,C).   *↳ red bacilli*
    6. Systemic spread often occurs and can involve any tissue; common sites include meninges (meningitis), cervical lymph nodes, kidneys (sterile pyuria), and lumbar vertebrae (Pott disease).   *→ @ base of brain*

CHRONIC OBSTRUCTIVE PULMONARY DISEASE

I. BASIC PRINCIPLES
A. Group of diseases characterized by airway obstruction; lung does not empty, and air is trapped.
    1. Volume of air that can be forcefully expired is decreased ($\downarrow$ FVC), especially during the first second of expiration ($\downarrow\downarrow$ FEV$_1$); results in $\downarrow$ FEV$_1$:FVC ratio
    2. Total lung capacity (TLC) is usually increased due to air trapping.

II. CHRONIC BRONCHITIS
A. Chronic productive cough lasting at least 3 months over a minimum of 2 years; highly associated with smoking
B. Characterized by hypertrophy of bronchial mucinous glands (Fig. 9.7)

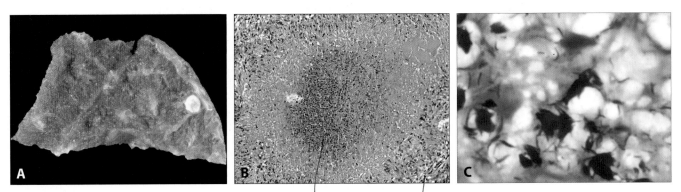

Fig. 9.6 Tuberculosis. **A**, Ghon complex. **B**, Caseating granuloma. **C**, AFB staining of *M tuberculosis*. (A, Courtesy of Yale Rosen, MD)

central necrosis   *epitheliod*   *red = ⊕ AFB*

1. Leads to increased thickness of mucus glands relative to bronchial wall thickness (Reid index increases to > 50%; normal is < 40%).

C. Clinical features
 1. Productive cough due to excessive mucus production
 2. Cyanosis ('blue bloaters')—Mucus plugs trap carbon dioxide; $\uparrow$ $Paco_2$ and $\downarrow$ Pao_2
 3. Increased risk of infection and cor pulmonale

III. EMPHYSEMA

A. Destruction of alveolar air sacs (Fig. 9.8)
 1. Loss of elastic recoil and collapse of airways during exhalation results in obstruction and air trapping.

B. Due to imbalance of proteases and antiproteases
 1. Inflammation in the lung normally leads to release of proteases by neutrophils and macrophages.
 2. α_1-antitrypsin (A1AT) neutralizes proteases.
 3. Excessive inflammation or lack of A1AT leads to destruction of the alveolar air sacs.

C. Smoking is the most common cause of emphysema.
 1. Pollutants in smoke lead to excessive inflammation and protease-mediated damage.
 2. Results in centriacinar emphysema that is most severe in the upper lobes

D. A1AT deficiency is a rare cause of emphysema.
 1. Lack of antiprotease leaves the air sacs vulnerable to protease-mediated damage.
 2. Results in panacinar emphysema that is most severe in the lower lobes
 3. Liver cirrhosis may also be present.
 i. A1AT deficiency is due to misfolding of the mutated protein.
 ii. Mutant A1AT accumulates in the endoplasmic reticulum of hepatocytes, resulting in liver damage.
 iii. Biopsy reveals pink, PAS-positive globules in hepatocytes (Fig. 9.9).
 4. Disease severity is based on the degree of A1AT deficiency.
 i. PiM is the normal allele; two copies are usually expressed (PiMM).
 ii. PiZ is the most common clinically relevant mutation; results in significantly low levels of circulating A1AT
 iii. PiMZ heterozygotes are usually asymptomatic with decreased circulating levels of A1AT; however, significant risk for emphysema with smoking exists.
 iv. PiZZ homozygotes are at significant risk for panacinar emphysema and cirrhosis.

E. Clinical features of emphysema include

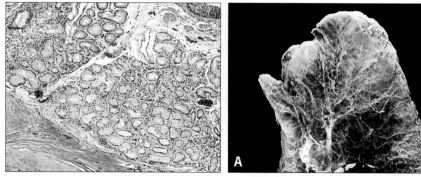

Fig. 9.7 Chronic bronchitis.

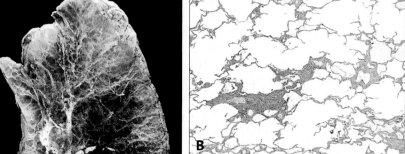

Fig. 9.8 Emphysema. **A,** Gross appearance. **B,** Microscopic appearance. (A, Courtesy of Yale Rosen, MD)

1. Dyspnea and cough with minimal sputum
2. Prolonged expiration with pursed lips ('pink-puffer')
3. Weight loss
4. Increased anterior-posterior diameter of chest ('barrel-chest,' Fig. 9.10)
5. Hypoxemia (due to destruction of capillaries in the alveolar sac) and cor pulmonale are late complications.

IV. **ASTHMA**
A. Reversible airway bronchoconstriction, most often due to allergic stimuli (atopic asthma)
B. Presents in childhood; often associated with allergic rhinitis, eczema, and a family history of atopy
C. Pathogenesis (type I hypersensitivity)
   1. Allergens induce T_H2 phenotype in $CD4^+$ T cells of genetically susceptible individuals.
   2. T_H2 cells secrete IL-4 (mediates class switch to IgE), IL-5 (attracts eosinophils), and IL-10 (stimulates T_H2 cells and inhibits T_H1).
   3. Reexposure to allergen leads to IgE-mediated activation of mast cells.
      i. Release of preformed histamine granules and generation of leukotrienes C4, D4, and E4 lead to bronchoconstriction, inflammation, and edema (early-phase reaction).
      ii. Inflammation, especially major basic protein derived from eosinophils, damages cells and perpetuates bronchoconstriction (late-phase reaction).
D. Clinical features are episodic and related to allergen exposure.
   1. Dyspnea and wheezing
   2. Productive cough, classically with spiral-shaped mucus plugs (Curschmann spirals) and eosinophil-derived crystals (Charcot-Leyden crystals, Fig. 9.11).
   3. Severe, unrelenting attack can result in status asthmaticus and death.
E. Asthma may also arise from nonallergic causes (non-atopic asthma) such as exercise, viral infection, aspirin (e.g., aspirin intolerant asthma), and occupational exposures.

V. **BRONCHIECTASIS**
A. Permanent dilatation of bronchioles and bronchi (Fig. 9.12); loss of airway tone results in air trapping.
B. Due to necrotizing inflammation with damage to airway walls. Causes include
   1. Cystic fibrosis
   2. Kartagener syndrome—inherited defect of the dynein arm, which is necessary for ciliary movement. Associated with sinusitis, infertility (poor motility of sperm), and situs inversus (position of major organs is reversed, e.g., heart is on right side of thorax)

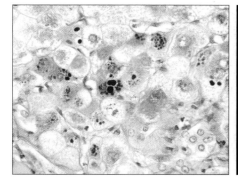
Fig. 9.9 A1AT accumulation in hepatocytes.

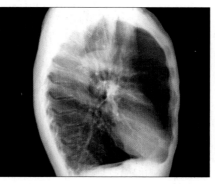
Fig. 9.10 Increased AP diameter, emphysema. (Courtesy of James Heilman, MD, Wikipedia)

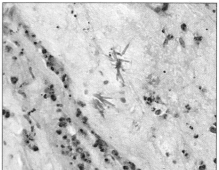
Fig. 9.11 Charcot-Leyden crystals, asthma.

   3. Tumor or foreign body
   4. Necrotizing infection
   5. Allergic bronchopulmonary aspergillosis—Hypersensitivity reaction to *Aspergillus* leads to chronic inflammatory damage; usually seen in individuals with asthma or cystic fibrosis
C. Clinical features
   1. Cough, dyspnea, and foul-smelling sputum
   2. Complications include hypoxemia with cor pulmonale and secondary (AA) amyloidosis.

RESTRICTIVE DISEASES

I. **BASIC PRINCIPLES**
   A. Characterized by restricted filling of the lung; $\downarrow$ TLC, $\downarrow$ FEV$_1$, and $\downarrow\downarrow$ FVC; FEV$_1$:FVC ratio is increased.
   B. Most commonly due to interstitial diseases of the lung; may also arise with chest wall abnormalities (e.g., massive obesity)

II. **IDIOPATHIC PULMONARY FIBROSIS**
   A. Fibrosis of lung interstitium (Fig. 9.13)
   B. Etiology is unknown. Likely related to cyclical lung injury; TGF-β from injured pneumocytes induces fibrosis.
      1. Secondary causes of interstitial fibrosis such as drugs (e.g., bleomycin and amiodarone) and radiation therapy must be excluded.
   C. Clinical features
      1. Progressive dyspnea and cough
      2. Fibrosis on lung CT; initially seen in subpleural patches, but eventually results in diffuse fibrosis with end-stage 'honeycomb' lung
      3. Treatment is lung transplantation.

III. **PNEUMOCONIOSES**
   A. Interstitial fibrosis due to occupational exposure; requires chronic exposure to small particles that are fibrogenic (Table 9.4)
      1. Alveolar macrophages engulf foreign particles and induce fibrosis.

IV. **SARCOIDOSIS**
   A. Systemic disease characterized by noncaseating granulomas in multiple organs; classically seen in African American females
   B. Etiology is unknown; likely due to CD4$^+$ helper T-cell response to an unknown antigen

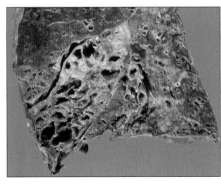

Fig. 9.12 Bronchiectasis. (Courtesy of Yale Rosen, MD)

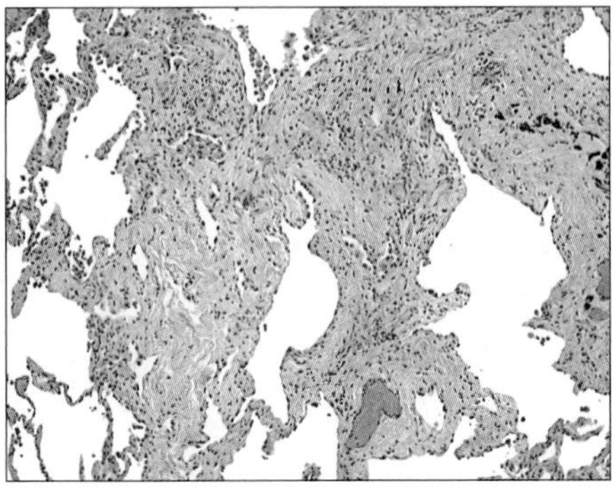

Fig. 9.13 Interstitial fibrosis, idiopathic pulmonary fibrosis.

Table 9.4: Summary of Pneumoconioses

ENTITY	EXPOSURE	PATHOLOGIC FINDINGS	COMMENTS
Coal Workers' Pneumoconiosis	Carbon dust; seen in coal miners	Massive exposure leads to diffuse fibrosis ('black lung'); associated with rheumatoid arthritis (Caplan syndrome)	Mild exposure to carbon (e.g., pollution) results in anthracosis (collections of carbon-laden macrophages); not clinically significant
Silicosis	Silica; seen in sandblasters and silica miners	Fibrotic nodules in upper lobes of the lung	Increased risk for TB; silica impairs phagolysosome formation by macrophages.
Berylliosis	Beryllium; seen in beryllium miners and workers in the aerospace industry	Noncaseating granulomas in the lung, hilar lymph nodes, and systemic organs	Increased risk for lung cancer
Asbestosis	Asbestos fibers; seen in construction workers, plumbers, and shipyard workers	Fibrosis of lung and pleura (plaques) with increased risk for lung carcinoma and mesothelioma; lung carcinoma is more common than mesothelioma in exposed individuals.	Lesions may contain long, golden-brown fibers with associated iron (asbestos bodies, Fig. 9.14), which confirm exposure to asbestos

C. Granulomas most commonly involve the hilar lymph nodes and lung (Fig. 9.15A), leading to restrictive lung disease.
   1. Characteristic stellate inclusions ('asteroid bodies') are often seen within giant cells of the granulomas (Fig. 9.15B).
D. Other commonly involved tissues include the uvea (uveitis), skin (cutaneous nodules or erythema nodosum), and salivary and lacrimal glands (mimics Sjögren syndrome); almost any tissue can be involved.
E. Clinical features
   1. Dyspnea or cough (most common presenting symptom)
   2. Elevated serum ACE
   3. Hypercalcemia (1-alpha hydroxylase activity of epithelioid histiocytes converts vitamin D to its active form)
   4. Treatment is steroids; often resolves spontaneously without treatment.

V. **HYPERSENSITIVITY PNEUMONITIS**
   A. Granulomatous reaction to inhaled organic antigens (e.g., pigeon breeder's lung)
   B. Presents with fever, cough, and dyspnea hours after exposure; resolves with removal of the exposure

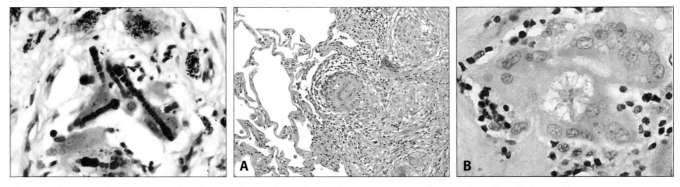

Fig. 9.14 Asbestos bodies. (Courtesy of Nephron, GNU-FDL v1.3)

Fig. 9.15 Sarcoidosis. **A**, Noncaseating granuloma involving lung. **B**, Asteroid body.

C. Chronic exposure leads to interstitial fibrosis.

PULMONARY HYPERTENSION

I. **BASIC PRINCIPLES**
    A. High pressure in the pulmonary circuit (mean arterial pressure > 25 mm Hg; normal is 10 mm Hg)
    B. Characterized by atherosclerosis of the pulmonary trunk, smooth muscle hypertrophy of pulmonary arteries, and intimal fibrosis; plexiform lesions are seen with severe, long-standing disease (Fig. 9.16).
    C. Leads to right ventricular hypertrophy with eventual cor pulmonale
    D. Presents with exertional dyspnea or right-sided heart failure
    E. Subclassified as primary or secondary based on etiology

II. **PRIMARY PULMONARY HYPERTENSION**
    A. Classically seen in young adult females
    B. Etiology is unknown; some familial forms are related to inactivating mutations of *BMPR2*, leading to proliferation of vascular smooth muscle.

III. **SECONDARY PULMONARY HYPERTENSION**
    A. Due to hypoxemia (e.g., COPD and interstitial lung disease) or increased volume in the pulmonary circuit (e.g., congenital heart disease); may also arise with recurrent pulmonary embolism

RESPIRATORY DISTRESS SYNDROMES

I. **ACUTE RESPIRATORY DISTRESS SYNDROME**
    A. Diffuse damage to the alveolar-capillary interface (diffuse alveolar damage)
    B. Leakage of protein-rich fluid leads to edema that combines with necrotic epithelial cells to form hyaline membranes in alveoli (Fig. 9.17A).
    C. Clinical features
        1. Hypoxemia and cyanosis with respiratory distress—due to thickened diffusion barrier and collapse of air sacs (increased surface tension)
        2. 'White-out' on chest x-ray (Fig. 9.17B)
    D. Secondary to a variety of disease processes including sepsis, infection, shock, trauma, aspiration, pancreatitis, DIC, hypersensitivity reactions, and drugs.
        1. Activation of neutrophils induces protease- and free radical-mediated damage of type I and II pneumocytes.
    E. Treatment
        1. Address underlying cause

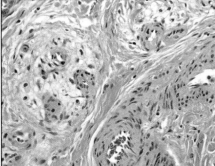

Fig. 9.16 Plexiform lesion, primary pulmonary hypertension.

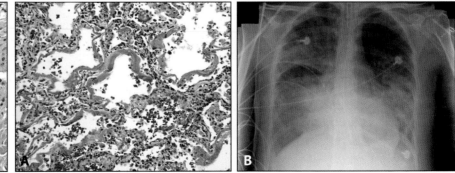

Fig. 9.17 ARDS. **A,** Hyaline membranes. **B,** 'White-out' of lung on x-ray. (B, Courtesy of Samir, GNU-FDL v1.2)

2. Ventilation with positive end-expiratory pressure (PEEP)

F. Recovery may be complicated by interstitial fibrosis; damage and loss of type II pneumocytes leads to scarring and fibrosis.

II. **NEONATAL RESPIRATORY DISTRESS SYNDROME**

A. Respiratory distress due to inadequate surfactant levels
    1. Surfactant is made by type II pneumocytes; phosphatidylcholine (lecithin) is the major component.
    2. Surfactant decreases surface tension in the lung, preventing collapse of alveolar air sacs after expiration.
    3. Lack of surfactant leads to collapse of air sacs and formation of hyaline membranes.

B. Associated with
    1. Prematurity—Surfactant production begins at 28 weeks; adequate levels are not reached until 34 weeks.
        i.   Amniotic fluid lecithin to sphingomyelin ratio is used to screen for lung maturity.
        ii. Phosphatidylcholine (lecithin) levels increase as surfactant is produced; sphingomyelin remains constant.
        iii. A ratio > 2 indicates adequate surfactant production.
    2. Caesarian section delivery—due to lack of stress-induced steroids; steroids increase synthesis of surfactant.
    3. Maternal diabetes—Insulin decreases surfactant production.

C. Clinical features
    1. Increasing respiratory effort after birth, tachypnea with use of accessory muscles, and grunting
    2. Hypoxemia with cyanosis
    3. Diffuse granularity of the lung ('ground-glass' appearance) on x-ray (Fig. 9.18)

D. Complications
    1. Hypoxemia increases the risk for persistence of patent ductus arteriosus and necrotizing enterocolitis.
    2. Supplemental oxygen increases the risk for free radical injury. Retinal injury leads to blindness; lung damage leads to bronchopulmonary dysplasia.

LUNG CANCER

I. **BASIC PRINCIPLES**

A. Most common cause of cancer mortality in the US; average age at presentation is 60 years.

B. Key risk factors are cigarette smoke, radon, and asbestos.
    1. Cigarette smoke contains over 60 carcinogens; 85% of lung cancer occurs in smokers.
        i.   Polycyclic aromatic hydrocarbons and arsenic are particularly mutagenic.
        ii. Cancer risk is directly related to the duration and amount of smoking ('pack-years').
    2. Radon is formed by radioactive decay of uranium, which is present in soil.
        i.   Accumulates in closed spaces such as basements
        ii. Responsible for most of the public exposure to ionizing radiation; 2nd most frequent cause of lung carcinoma in US
        iii. Increased risk of lung cancer is also seen in uranium miners.

C. Presenting symptoms are nonspecific (e.g., cough, weight loss, hemoptysis, and postobstructive pneumonia).

D. Imaging often reveals a solitary nodule ('coin-lesion'); biopsy is necessary for a diagnosis of cancer.

    1. Benign lesions, which often occur in younger patients, can also produce a 'coin-lesion.' Examples include

        i. Granuloma—often due to TB or fungus (especially *Histoplasma* in the Midwest)

        ii. Bronchial hamartoma—benign tumor composed of lung tissue and cartilage; often calcified on imaging

E. Lung carcinoma is classically divided into 2 categories (Table 9.5).

    1. Small cell carcinoma (15%)—usually not amenable to surgical resection (treated with chemotherapy)

    2. Non-small cell carcinoma (85%)—treated upfront with surgical resection (does not respond well to chemotherapy); subtypes include adenocarcinoma (40%), squamous cell carcinoma (30%), large cell carcinoma (10%), and carcinoid tumor (5%).

F. TNM staging

    1. T—Tumor size and local extension

        i. Pleural involvement is classically seen with adenocarcinoma.

        ii. Obstruction of SVC leads to distended head and neck veins with edema and blue discoloration of arms and face (superior vena cava syndrome).

        iii. Involvement of recurrent laryngeal (hoarseness) or phrenic (diaphragmatic paralysis) nerve

Table 9.5: Cancers of the Lung

CANCER	CHARACTERISTIC HISTOLOGY	ASSOCIATION	LOCATION	COMMENT
Small cell carcinoma	Poorly differentiated small cells (Fig. 9.19); arises from neuroendocrine (Kulchitsky) cells	Male smokers	Central	Rapid growth and early metastasis; may produce ADH or ACTH or cause Eaton-Lambert syndrome (paraneoplastic syndromes)
Squamous cell carcinoma	Keratin pearls or intercellular bridges (Fig. 9.20A,B)	Most common tumor in male smokers	Central (Fig. 9.20C)	May produce PTHrP
Adenocarcinoma	Glands or mucin (Fig. 9.21A)	Most common tumor in nonsmokers and female smokers	Peripheral (Fig. 9.21B)	
Large cell Carcinoma	Poorly differentiated large cells (no keratin pearls, intercellular bridges, glands, or mucin)	Smoking	Central or peripheral	Poor prognosis
Bronchioloalveolar carcinoma	Columnar cells that grow along preexisting bronchioles and alveoli (Fig. 9.22); arises from Clara cells	Not related to smoking	Peripheral	May present with pneumonia-like consolidation on imaging; excellent prognosis
Carcinoid tumor	Well differentiated neuroendocrine cells; chromogranin positive (Fig. 9.23A,B)	Not related to smoking	Central or peripheral; when central, classically forms a polyp-like mass in the bronchus (Fig. 9.23C)	Low-grade malignancy; rarely, can cause carcinoid syndrome
Metastasis to lung	Most common sources are breast and colon carcinoma.		Multiple 'cannon-ball' nodules on imaging	More common than primary tumors

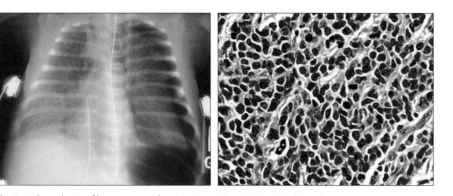

Fig. 9.18 Granularity of lung, neonatal respiratory distress syndrome. (Published with permission from LearningRadiology.com)

Fig. 9.19 Small cell carcinoma.

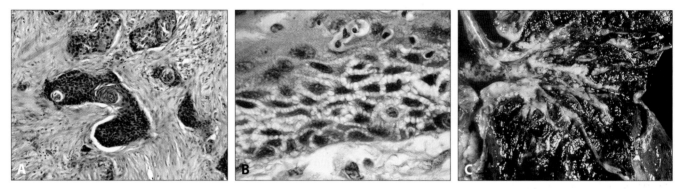

Fig. 9.20 Squamous cell carcinoma. **A**, Keratin pearls. **B**, Intercellular bridges. **C**, Central location. (B, Courtesy Thomas Krausz, MD. C, Courtesy of Yale Rosen, MD)

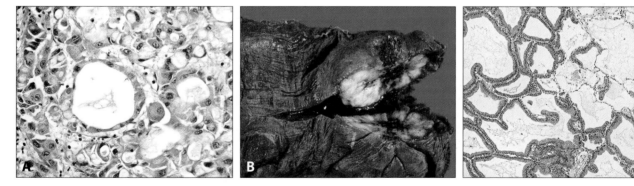

Fig. 9.21 Adenocarcinoma. **A**, Gland formation and mucin production. **B**, Peripheral location. (B, Courtesy of Thomas Krausz, MD)

Fig. 9.22 Bronchioloalveolar carcinoma.

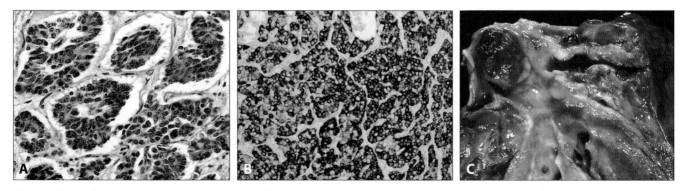

Fig. 9.23 Carcinoid tumor. **A**, Microscopic appearance. **B**, Chromogranin expression by immunohistochemistry. **C**, Polyp-like growth in the bronchus. (C, Courtesy of Yale Rosen, MD)

  iv. Compression of sympathetic chain leads to Horner syndrome characterized by ptosis (drooping eyelid), miosis (pinpoint pupil), and anhidrosis (no sweating); usually due to an apical (Pancoast) tumor

 2. N—spread to regional lymph nodes (hilar and mediastinal)

 3. M—unique site of distant metastasis is the adrenal gland.

 4. Overall, 15% 5-year survival; often presents late due to the absence of an effective screening method

PLEURA

I. **PNEUMOTHORAX**

 A. Accumulation of air in the pleural space

 B. Spontaneous pneumothorax is due to rupture of an emphysematous bleb; seen in young adults

  1. Results in collapse of a portion of the lung (Fig. 9.24); trachea shifts to the side of collapse.

 C. Tension pneumothorax arises with penetrating chest wall injury.

  1. Air enters the pleural space, but cannot exit; trachea is pushed opposite to the side of injury.

  2. Medical emergency; treated with insertion of a chest tube

II. **MESOTHELIOMA**

 A. Malignant neoplasm of mesothelial cells; highly associated with occupational exposure to asbestos

 B. Presents with recurrent pleural effusions, dyspnea, and chest pain; tumor encases the lung (Fig. 9.25).

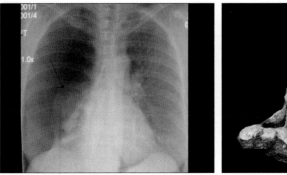

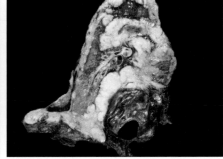

Fig. 9.24 Spontaneous pneumothorax. (Courtesy of James Heilman, MD, Wikipedia.)

Fig. 9.25 Mesothelioma. (Courtesy of Jamie Steinmetz, MD)

Gastrointestinal Pathology

10

ORAL CAVITY

I. **CLEFT LIP AND PALATE**
   A. Full-thickness defect of lip or palate (Fig. 10.1)
   B. Due to failure of facial prominences to fuse
      1. During early pregnancy, facial prominences (one from superior, two from the sides, and two from inferior) grow and fuse together to form the face.
   C. Cleft lip and palate usually occur together; isolated cleft lip or palate is less common.

II. **APHTHOUS ULCER**
   A. Painful, superficial ulceration of the oral mucosa (Fig. 10.2)
   B. Arises in relation to stress and resolves spontaneously, but often recurs
   C. Characterized by a grayish base surrounded by erythema

III. **BEHÇET SYNDROME**
   A. Recurrent aphthous ulcers, genital ulcers, and uveitis
   B. Due to immune complex vasculitis involving small vessels
   C. Can be seen after viral infection, but etiology is unknown

IV. **ORAL HERPES**
   A. Vesicles involving oral mucosa that rupture, resulting in shallow, painful, red ulcers
   B. Usually due to HSV-1
   C. Primary infection occurs in childhood; lesions heal, but virus remains dormant in ganglia of the trigeminal nerve.
   D. Stress and sunlight cause reactivation of the virus, leading to vesicles that often arise on the lips (cold sore, Fig. 10.3).

V. **SQUAMOUS CELL CARCINOMA**
   A. Malignant neoplasm of squamous cells lining the oral mucosa
   B. Tobacco and alcohol are major risk factors.
   C. Floor of mouth is the most common location.
   D. Oral leukoplakia and erythroplakia are precursor lesions.
      1. Leukoplakia is a white plaque that cannot be scraped away; often represents squamous cell dysplasia
      2. Leukoplakia is distinct from oral candidiasis (thrush) and hairy leukoplakia.
         i. Oral candidiasis is a white deposit on the tongue, which is *easily* scraped away (Fig. 10.4); usually seen in immunocompromised states
         ii. Hairy leukoplakia is a white, rough ('hairy') patch that arises on the lateral tongue. It is usually seen in immunocompromised individuals (e.g., AIDS) and is due to EBV-induced squamous cell hyperplasia; not pre-malignant
      3. Erythroplakia (red plaque) represents vascularized leukoplakia and is highly suggestive of squamous cell dysplasia.
      4. Erythroplakia and leukoplakia are often biopsied to rule out carcinoma.

SALIVARY GLAND

I. **BASIC PRINCIPLES**
   A. Salivary glands are exocrine glands that secrete saliva.
   B. Divided into major (parotid, submandibular, and sublingual glands) and minor glands (hundreds of microscopic glands distributed throughout the oral mucosa)

II. **MUMPS**
   A. Infection with mumps virus resulting in bilateral inflamed parotid glands
   B. Orchitis, pancreatitis, and aseptic meningitis may also be present.
      1. Serum amylase is increased due to salivary gland or pancreatic involvement.
      2. Orchitis carries risk of sterility, especially in teenagers.

III. **SIALADENITIS**
   A. Inflammation of the salivary gland
   B. Most commonly due to an obstructing stone (sialolithiasis) leading to *Staphylococcus aureus* infection; usually unilateral

IV. **PLEOMORPHIC ADENOMA**
   A. Benign tumor composed of stromal (e.g., cartilage) and epithelial tissue; most common tumor of the salivary gland
   B. Usually arises in parotid; presents as a mobile, painless, circumscribed mass at the angle of the jaw
   C. High rate of recurrence; extension of small islands of tumor through tumor capsule often leads to incomplete resection (Fig. 10.5).
   D. Rarely may transform into carcinoma, which presents with signs of facial nerve damage (facial nerve runs through parotid gland)

V. **WARTHIN TUMOR**
   A. Benign cystic tumor with abundant lymphocytes and germinal centers (lymph node-like stroma); 2nd most common tumor of the salivary gland
   B. Almost always arises in the parotid

VI. **MUCOEPIDERMOID CARCINOMA**
   A. Malignant tumor composed of mucinous and squamous cells; most common malignant tumor of the salivary gland
   B. Usually arises in the parotid; commonly involves the facial nerve

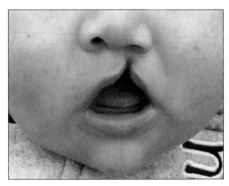

Fig. 10.1 Cleft lip and palate. (Courtesy of James Heilman, MD, Wikipedia)

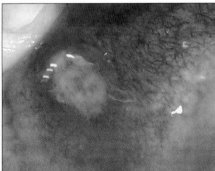

Fig. 10.2 Aphthous ulcer. (Reproduced from wikipedia.org, CCBY-SA 3.0)

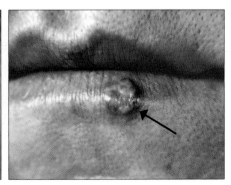

Fig. 10.3 Cold sore. (Courtesy of Dr. Herrmann, CDC)

ESOPHAGUS

I. **TRACHEOESOPHAGEAL FISTULA**
   A. Congenital defect resulting in a connection between the esophagus and trachea
   B. Most common variant consists of proximal esophageal atresia with the distal esophagus arising from the trachea (Fig. 10.6).
      1. Presents with vomiting, polyhydramnios, abdominal distension, and aspiration

II. **ESOPHAGEAL WEB**
   A. Thin protrusion of esophageal mucosa, most often in the upper esophagus
   B. Presents with dysphagia for poorly chewed food
   C. Increased risk for esophageal squamous cell carcinoma
   D. Plummer-Vinson syndrome is characterized by severe iron deficiency anemia, esophageal web, and beefy-red tongue due to atrophic glossitis.

III. **ZENKER DIVERTICULUM**
   A. Outpouching of pharyngeal mucosa through an acquired defect in the muscular wall (false diverticulum)
   B. Arises above the upper esophageal sphincter at the junction of the esophagus and pharynx
   C. Presents with dysphagia, obstruction, and halitosis (bad breath)

IV. **MALLORY-WEISS SYNDROME**
   A. Longitudinal laceration of mucosa at the gastroesophageal (GE) junction
   B. Caused by severe vomiting, usually due to alcoholism or bulimia
   C. Presents with painful hematemesis
   D. Risk of Boerhaave syndrome—rupture of esophagus leading to air in the mediastinum and subcutaneous emphysema

V. **ESOPHAGEAL VARICES**
   A. Dilated submucosal veins in the lower esophagus
   B. Arise secondary to portal hypertension
      1. Distal esophageal vein normally drains into the portal vein via the left gastric vein.
      2. In portal hypertension, the left gastric vein backs up into the esophageal vein, resulting in dilation (varices).
   C. Asymptomatic, but risk of rupture exists
      1. Presents with painless hematemesis
      2. Most common cause of death in cirrhosis

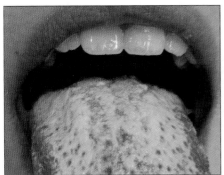

Fig. 10.4 Oral candidiasis. (Courtesy of James Heilman, MD, Wikipedia)

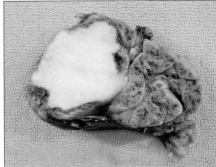

Fig. 10.5 Pleomorphic adenoma. (Courtesy of Bulent Celasun, MD)

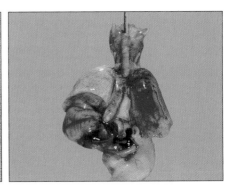

Fig. 10.6 Tracheoesophageal fistula. (Courtesy of humpath.com)

VI. ACHALASIA

A. Disordered esophageal motility with inability to relax the lower esophageal sphincter (LES)

B. Due to damaged ganglion cells in the myenteric plexus

    1. Ganglion cells of myenteric plexus are located between the inner circular and outer longitudinal layers of the muscularis propria and are important for regulating bowel motility and relaxing the LES.

    2. Damage to ganglion cells can be idiopathic or secondary to a known insult (e.g., *Trypanosoma cruzi* infection in Chagas disease).

C. Clinical features

    1. Dysphagia for solids and liquids

    2. Putrid breath

    3. High LES pressure on esophageal manometry

    4. 'Bird-beak' sign on barium swallow study (Fig. 10.7)

    5. Increased risk for esophageal squamous cell carcinoma

VII. GASTROESOPHAGEAL REFLUX DISEASE (GERD)

A. Reflux of acid from the stomach due to reduced LES tone

B. Risk factors include alcohol, tobacco, obesity, fat-rich diet, caffeine, and hiatal hernia.

C. Clinical features

    1. Heartburn (mimics cardiac chest pain)

    2. Asthma (adult-onset) and cough

    3. Damage to enamel of teeth

    4. Ulceration with stricture and Barrett esophagus are late complications.

VIII. BARRETT ESOPHAGUS

A. Metaplasia of the lower esophageal mucosa from stratified squamous epithelium to nonciliated columnar epithelium with goblet cells (Fig. 10.8); seen in 10% of patients with GERD

    1. Response of lower esophageal stem cells to acidic stress

B. May progress to dysplasia and adenocarcinoma

IX. ESOPHAGEAL CARCINOMA

A. Subclassified as adenocarcinoma or squamous cell carcinoma

B. Adenocarcinoma is a malignant proliferation of glands; most common type of esophageal carcinoma in the West

    1. Arises from preexisting Barrett esophagus; usually involves the lower one-third of the esophagus

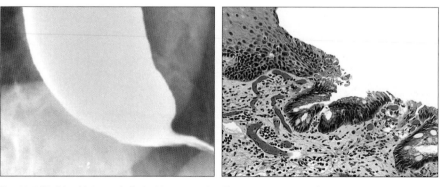

Fig. 10.7 'Bird-beak' sign, achalasia. (Courtesy of F. Farrokhi, MD and M. Vaezi, MD)   **Fig. 10.8** Barrett esophagus.

C. Squamous cell carcinoma is a malignant proliferation of squamous cells; most common esophageal cancer worldwide

    1. Usually arises in upper or middle third of the esophagus; major risk factors include

        i. Alcohol and tobacco (most common causes)

        ii. Very hot tea

        iii. Achalasia

        iv. Esophageal web (e.g., Plummer-Vinson syndrome)

        v. Esophageal injury (e.g., lye ingestion)

D. Esophageal carcinoma presents late (poor prognosis).

    1. Symptoms include progressive dysphagia (solids to liquids), weight loss, pain, and hematemesis.

    2. Squamous cell carcinoma may additionally present with hoarse voice (recurrent laryngeal nerve involvement) and cough (tracheal involvement).

E. Location of lymph node spread depends on the level of the esophagus that is involved.

    1. Upper 1/3—cervical nodes

    2. Middle 1/3—mediastinal or tracheobronchial nodes

    3. Lower 1/3—celiac and gastric nodes

STOMACH

I. **GASTROSCHISIS**

    A. Congenital malformation of the anterior abdominal wall leading to exposure of abdominal contents (Fig. 10.9)

II. **OMPHALOCELE**

    A. Persistent herniation of bowel into umbilical cord

    B. Due to failure of herniated intestines to return to the body cavity during development

        1. Contents are covered by peritoneum and amnion of the umbilical cord (Fig. 10.10).

III. **PYLORIC STENOSIS**

    A. Congenital hypertrophy of pyloric smooth muscle; more common in males

    B. Classically presents two weeks after birth as

        1. Projectile nonbilious vomiting

        2. Visible peristalsis

        3. Olive-like mass in the abdomen

    C. Treatment is myotomy.

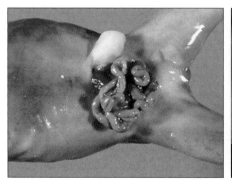

Fig. 10.9 Gastroschisis. (Courtesy of humpath.com)

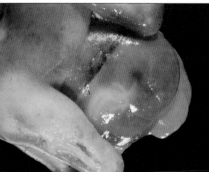

Fig. 10.10 Omphalocele. (Courtesy of J.T. Stocker, MD)

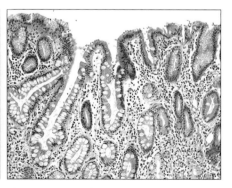

Fig. 10.11 Intestinal metaplasia, chronic gastritis.

IV. **ACUTE GASTRITIS**
   A. Acidic damage to the stomach mucosa
   B. Due to imbalance between mucosal defenses and acidic environment
      1. Defenses include mucin layer produced by foveolar cells, bicarbonate secretion by surface epithelium, and normal blood supply (provides nutrients and picks up leaked acid).
   C. Risk factors
      1. Severe burn (Curling ulcer)—Hypovolemia leads to decreased blood supply.
      2. NSAIDs (decreased PGE_2)
      3. Heavy alcohol consumption
      4. Chemotherapy
      5. Increased intracranial pressure (Cushing ulcer)—Increased stimulation of vagus nerve leads to increased acid production.
      6. Shock—Multiple (stress) ulcers may be seen in ICU patients.
   D. Acid damage results in superficial inflammation, erosion (loss of superficial epithelium), or ulcer (loss of mucosal layer).

V. **CHRONIC GASTRITIS**
   A. Chronic inflammation of stomach mucosa
   B. Divided into two types based on underlying etiology: chronic autoimmune gastritis and chronic *H pylori* gastritis
   C. Chronic autoimmune gastritis is due to autoimmune destruction of gastric parietal cells, which are located in the stomach body and fundus.
      1. Associated with antibodies against parietal cells and/or intrinsic factor; useful for diagnosis, but pathogenesis is mediated by T cells (type IV hypersensitivity)
      2. Clinical features
         i. Atrophy of mucosa with intestinal metaplasia (Fig. 10.11)
         ii. Achlorhydria with increased gastrin levels and antral G-cell hyperplasia
         iii. Megaloblastic (pernicious) anemia due to lack of intrinsic factor
         iv. Increased risk for gastric adenocarcinoma (intestinal type)
   D. Chronic *H pylori* gastritis is due to *H pylori*-induced acute and chronic inflammation; most common form of gastritis (90%)
      1. *H pylori* ureases and proteases along with inflammation weaken mucosal defenses; antrum is the most common site (Fig. 10.12).
      2. Presents with epigastric abdominal pain; increased risk for ulceration (peptic ulcer disease), gastric adenocarcinoma (intestinal type), and MALT lymphoma
      3. Treatment involves triple therapy.
         i. Resolves gastritis/ulcer and reverses intestinal metaplasia
         ii. Negative urea breath test and lack of stool antigen confirm eradication of *H pylori*.

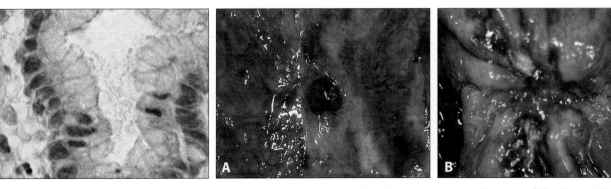

Fig. 10.12 *H pylori*. (Courtesy of Ed Uthman, MD)   **Fig. 10.13** Gastric ulcer. **A**, Peptic ulcer disease. **B**, Carcinoma. (Courtesy of Aliya Husain, MD)

VI. PEPTIC ULCER DISEASE

A. Solitary mucosal ulcer involving proximal duodenum (90%) or distal stomach (10%)

B. Duodenal ulcer is almost always due to *H pylori* (> 95%); rarely, may be due to ZE syndrome
   1. Presents with epigastric pain that improves with meals
   2. Diagnostic endoscopic biopsy shows ulcer with hypertrophy of Brunner glands.
   3. Usually arises in anterior duodenum; when present in posterior duodenum, rupture may lead to bleeding from the gastroduodenal artery or acute pancreatitis

C. Gastric ulcer is usually due to *H pylori* (75%); other causes include NSAIDs and bile reflux.
   1. Presents with epigastric pain that worsens with meals
   2. Ulcer is usually located on the lesser curvature of the antrum.
   3. Rupture carries risk of bleeding from left gastric artery.

D. Differential diagnosis of ulcers includes carcinoma.
   1. Duodenal ulcers are almost never malignant (duodenal carcinoma is extremely rare).
   2. Gastric ulcers can be caused by gastric carcinoma (intestinal subtype).
      i. Benign peptic ulcers are usually small (< 3 cm), sharply demarcated ("punched-out"), and surrounded by radiating folds of mucosa (Fig. 10.13A).
      ii. Malignant ulcers are large and irregular with heaped up margins (Fig. 10.13B)
      iii. Biopsy is required for definitive diagnosis.

VII. GASTRIC CARCINOMA

A. Malignant proliferation of surface epithelial cells (adenocarcinoma)

B. Subclassified into intestinal and diffuse types

C. Intestinal type (more common) presents as a large, irregular ulcer with heaped up margins; most commonly involves the lesser curvature of the antrum (similar to gastric ulcer)
   1. Risk factors include intestinal metaplasia (e.g., due to *H pylori* and autoimmune gastritis), nitrosamines in smoked foods (Japan), and blood type A.

D. Diffuse type is characterized by signet ring cells that diffusely infiltrate the gastric wall (Fig. 10.14B); desmoplasia results in thickening of stomach wall (linitis plastica, Fig. 10.14A).
   1. Not associated with *H pylori*, intestinal metaplasia, or nitrosamines

E. Gastric carcinoma presents late with weight loss, abdominal pain, anemia, and early satiety; rarely presents as acanthosis nigricans or Leser-Trélat sign

F. Spread to lymph nodes can involve the left supraclavicular node (Virchow node).

G. Distant metastasis most commonly involves liver; other sites include
   1. Periumbilical region (Sister Mary Joseph nodule); seen with intestinal type

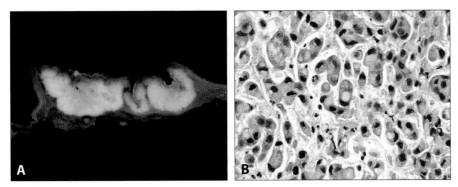

Fig. 10.14 Gastric carcinoma, diffuse type. **A**, Linitis plastica. **B**, Signet-ring cells. (A, Courtesy of Ed Uthman, MD)

2. Bilateral ovaries (Krukenberg tumor); seen with diffuse type

SMALL BOWEL

I. **DUODENAL ATRESIA**
    A. Congenital failure of duodenum to canalize; associated with Down syndrome
    B. Clinical features
        1. Polyhydramnios
        2. Distension of stomach and blind loop of duodenum ('double bubble' sign, Fig. 10.15)
        3. Bilious vomiting

II. **MECKEL DIVERTICULUM**
    A. Outpouching of all three layers of the bowel wall (true diverticulum, Fig. 10.16)
    B. Arises due to failure of the vitelline duct to involute
    C. 'Rule of 2s'
        1. Seen in 2% of the population (most common congenital anomaly of the GI tract)
        2. 2 inches long and located in the small bowel within 2 feet of the ileocecal valve
        3. Can present during the first 2 years of life with bleeding (due to heterotopic gastric mucosa), volvulus, intussusception, or obstruction (mimics appendicitis); however, most cases are asymptomatic.

III. **VOLVULUS**
    A. Twisting of bowel along its mesentery
    B. Results in obstruction and disruption of the blood supply with infarction (Fig. 10.17)
    C. Most common locations are sigmoid colon (elderly) and cecum (young adults).

IV. **INTUSSUSCEPTION**
    A. Telescoping of proximal segment of bowel forward into distal segment
        1. Telescoped segment is pulled forward by peristalsis, resulting in obstruction and disruption of blood supply with infarction.
    B. Associated with a leading edge (focus of traction)
        1. In children, the most common cause is lymphoid hyperplasia (e.g., due to rotavirus); usually arises in the terminal ileum, leading to intussusception into the cecum
        2. In adults, the most common cause is tumor.

V. **SMALL BOWEL INFARCTION**
    A. Small bowel is highly susceptible to ischemic injury.

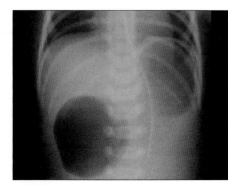

Fig. 10.15 'Double bubble' sign, duodenal atresia. (Courtesy of Auckland District Health Board)

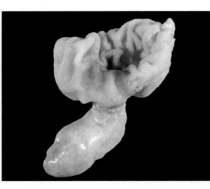

Fig. 10.16 Meckel diverticulum. (Courtesy of humpath.com)

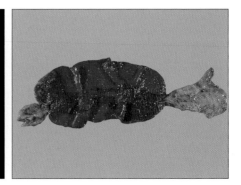

Fig. 10.17 Infarction due to volvulus. (Courtesy of humpath.com)

1. Transmural infarction occurs with thrombosis/embolism of the superior mesenteric artery or thrombosis of the mesenteric vein.
2. Mucosal infarction occurs with marked hypotension.

B. Clinical features include abdominal pain, bloody diarrhea, and decreased bowel sounds.

VI. LACTOSE INTOLERANCE

A. Decreased function of the lactase enzyme found in the brush border of enterocytes
   1. Lactase normally breaks down lactose into glucose and galactose.
B. Presents with abdominal distension and diarrhea upon consumption of milk products; undigested lactose is osmotically active.
C. Deficiency may be congenital (rare autosomal recessive disorder) or acquired (often develops in late childhood); temporary deficiency is seen after small bowel infection (lactase is highly susceptible to injury).

VII. CELIAC DISEASE

A. Immune-mediated damage of small bowel villi due to gluten exposure; associated with HLA-DQ2 and DQ8
B. Gluten is present in wheat and grains; its most pathogenic component is gliadin.
   1. Once absorbed, gliadin is deamidated by tissue transglutaminase (tTG).
   2. Deamidated gliadin is presented by antigen presenting cells via MHC class II.
   3. Helper T cells mediate tissue damage.
C. Clinical presentation
   1. Children classically present with abdominal distension, diarrhea, and failure to thrive.
   2. Adults classically present with chronic diarrhea and bloating.
   3. Small, herpes-like vesicles may arise on skin (dermatitis herpetiformis). Due to IgA deposition at the tips of dermal papillae; resolves with gluten-free diet
D. Laboratory findings
   1. IgA antibodies against endomysium, tTG, or gliadin; IgG antibodies are also present and are useful for diagnosis in individuals with IgA deficiency (increased incidence of IgA deficiency is seen in celiac disease).
   2. Duodenal biopsy reveals flattening of villi, hyperplasia of crypts, and increased intraepithelial lymphocytes (Fig. 10.18). Damage is most prominent in the duodenum; jejunum and ileum are less involved.
E. Symptoms resolve with gluten-free diet.
   1. Small bowel carcinoma and T-cell lymphoma are late complications that present as refractory disease despite good dietary control.

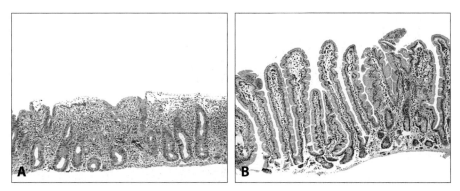

Fig. 10.18 Celiac disease. **A**, Flattened villi. **B**, Normal villi for comparison.

VIII. **TROPICAL SPRUE**
  A. Damage to small bowel villi due to an unknown organism resulting in malabsorption
  B. Similar to celiac disease except
    1. Occurs in tropical regions (e.g., Caribbean)
    2. Arises after infectious diarrhea and responds to antibiotics
    3. Damage is most prominent in jejunum and ileum (secondary vitamin B12 or folate deficiency may ensue); duodenum is less commonly involved.

IX. **WHIPPLE DISEASE**
  A. Systemic tissue damage characterized by macrophages loaded with *Tropheryma whippelii* organisms; partially destroyed organisms are present in macrophage lysosomes (positive for PAS).
  B. Classic site of involvement is the small bowel lamina propria (Fig. 10.19).
    1. Macrophages compress lacteals.
    2. Chylomicrons cannot be transferred from enterocytes to lymphatics.
    3. Results in fat malabsorption and steatorrhea
  C. Other common sites of involvement include synovium of joints (arthritis), cardiac valves, lymph nodes, and CNS.

X. **ABETALIPOPROTEINEMIA**
  A. Autosomal recessive deficiency of apolipoprotein B-48 and B-100
  B. Clinical features
    1. Malabsorption—due to defective chylomicron formation (requires B-48)
    2. Absent plasma VLDL and LDL (require B-100)

XI. **CARCINOID TUMOR**
  A. Malignant proliferation of neuroendocrine cells; low-grade malignancy
    1. Tumor cells contain neurosecretory granules that are positive for chromogranin.
  B. Can arise anywhere along the gut; small bowel is the most common site.
    1. Grows as a submucosal polyp-like nodule (Fig. 10.20)
  C. Often secretes serotonin
    1. Serotonin is released into the portal circulation and metabolized by liver monoamine oxidase (MAO) into 5-HIAA.
    2. 5-HIAA is excreted in the urine.
  D. Metastasis of carcinoid tumor to the liver allows serotonin to bypass liver metabolism.
    1. Serotonin is released into the hepatic vein and leaks into systemic circulation via hepato-systemic shunts, resulting in carcinoid syndrome and carcinoid heart disease.

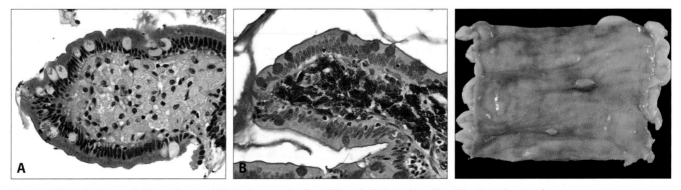

Fig. 10.19 Whipple disease. **A,** Macrophages within lamina propria of small bowel villi. **B,** *T whippelii* organisms highlighted by PAS stain.   **Fig. 10.20** Carcinoid tumor.

2. Carcinoid syndrome is characterized by bronchospasm, diarrhea, and flushing of skin; symptoms can be triggered by alcohol or emotional stress, which stimulate serotonin release from the tumor.

3. Carcinoid heart disease is characterized by right-sided valvular fibrosis (increased collagen) leading to tricuspid regurgitation and pulmonary valve stenosis; left-sided valvular lesions are not seen due to presence of monoamine oxidase (metabolizes serotonin) in the lung.

APPENDIX

I. **ACUTE APPENDICITIS**
   A. Acute inflammation of the appendix; most common cause of acute abdomen
   B. Related to obstruction of the appendix by lymphoid hyperplasia (children) or a fecalith (adults)
   C. Clinical features include
      1. Periumbilical pain, fever, and nausea; pain eventually localizes to right lower quadrant (McBurney point).
      2. Rupture results in peritonitis that presents with guarding and rebound tenderness.
      3. Periappendiceal abscess is a common complication.

INFLAMMATORY BOWEL DISEASE

I. **BASIC PRINCIPLES**
   A. Chronic, relapsing inflammation of bowel
   B. Possibly due to abnormal immune response to enteric flora
   C. Classically presents in young women (teens to 30s) as recurrent bouts of bloody diarrhea and abdominal pain
      1. More prevalent in the West, particularly in Caucasians and Eastern European Jews
   D. Diagnosis of exclusion; symptoms mimic other causes of bowel inflammation (e.g., infection).
   E. Subclassified as ulcerative colitis or Crohn disease (Table 10.1)

COLON

I. **HIRSCHSPRUNG DISEASE**
   A. Defective relaxation and peristalsis of rectum and distal sigmoid colon
      1. Associated with Down syndrome
   B. Due to congenital failure of ganglion cells (neural crest-derived) to descend into myenteric and submucosal plexus
      1. Myenteric (Auerbach) plexus is located between the inner circular and outer longitudinal muscle layers of the muscularis propria and regulates motility.
      2. Submucosal (Meissner) plexus is located in the submucosa and regulates blood flow, secretions, and absorption.
   C. Clinical features are based on obstruction.
      1. Failure to pass meconium
      2. Empty rectal vault on digital rectal exam
      3. Massive dilatation (megacolon) of bowel proximal to obstruction with risk for rupture
   D. Rectal suction biopsy reveals lack of ganglion cells.
   E. Treatment involves resection of the involved bowel; ganglion cells are present in the bowel proximal to the diseased segment.

Table 10.1: Main Features of Ulcerative Colitis and Crohn Disease

	ULCERATIVE COLITIS (UC)	CROHN DISEASE
Wall Involvement	Mucosal and submucosal ulcers	Full-thickness inflammation with knife-like fissures
Location	Begins in rectum and can extend proximally up to the cecum (involvement is continuous, Fig. 10.21A); remainder of the GI tract is unaffected.	Anywhere from mouth to anus with skip lesions; terminal ileum is the most common site, rectum is least common.
Symptoms	Left lower quadrant pain (rectum) with bloody diarrhea	Right lower quadrant pain (ileum) with non-bloody diarrhea
Inflammation	Crypt abscesses with neutrophils (Fig. 10.21B)	Lymphoid aggregates with granulomas (40% of cases)
Gross Appearance	Pseudopolyps; loss of haustra ('lead pipe' sign on imaging, Fig. 10.21C)	Cobblestone mucosa (Fig. 10.22A), creeping fat, and strictures ('string-sign' on imaging, Fig. 10.22B)
Complications	Toxic megacolon and carcinoma (risk is based on extent of colonic involvement and duration of disease; generally not a concern until > 10 years of disease)	Malabsorption with nutritional deficiency, calcium oxalate nephrolithiasis, fistula formation, and carcinoma, if colonic disease is present
Associations	Primary sclerosing cholangitis, p-ANCA positivity, and joint problems such as ankylosing spondylitis, sacroiliitis, and migratory polyarthritis	Erythema nodosum and uveitis
Smoking	Protects against UC	Increases risk for Crohn disease

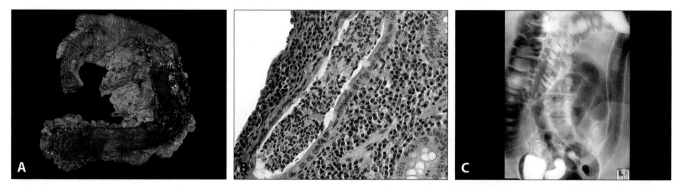

Fig. 10.21 Ulcerative colitis. A, Gross appearance. B, Crypt abscess. C, 'Lead pipe' sign (A, Courtesy of Jamie Steinmetz, MD. C, Published with permission from LearningRadiology.com)

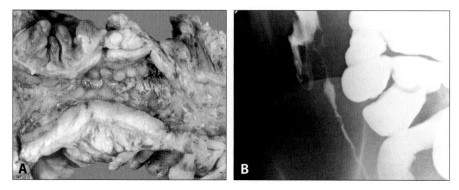

Fig. 10.22 Crohn disease. A, Cobblestone mucosa with stricture. B, 'String' sign. (A, Courtesy of humpath.com. B, Published with permission from LearningRadiology.com)

II. COLONIC DIVERTICULA

A. Outpouchings of mucosa and submucosa through the muscularis propria (Fig. 10.23, false diverticulum)

B. Related to wall stress

   1. Associated with constipation, straining, and low-fiber diet; commonly seen in older adults (risk increases with age)

   2. Arise where the vasa recta traverse the muscularis propria (weak point in colonic wall); sigmoid colon is the most common location.

C. Usually asymptomatic; complications include

   1. Rectal bleeding (hematochezia)

   2. Diverticulitis—due to obstructing fecal material; presents with appendicitis-like symptoms in the *left* lower quadrant

   3. Fistula—Inflamed diverticulum ruptures and attaches to a local structure. Colovesicular fistula presents with air (or stool) in urine.

III. ANGIODYSPLASIA

A. Acquired malformation of mucosal and submucosal capillary beds

B. Usually arises in the cecum and right colon due to high wall tension

C. Rupture classically presents as hematochezia in an older adult.

IV. HEREDITARY HEMORRHAGIC TELANGIECTASIA

A. Autosomal dominant disorder resulting in thin-walled blood vessels, especially in the mouth and GI tract (Fig. 10.24)

B. Rupture presents as bleeding.

V. ISCHEMIC COLITIS

A. Ischemic damage to the colon, usually at the splenic flexure (watershed area of superior mesenteric artery [SMA])

B. Atherosclerosis of SMA is the most common cause.

C. Presents with postprandial pain and weight loss; infarction results in pain and bloody diarrhea.

VI. IRRITABLE BOWEL SYNDROME

A. Relapsing abdominal pain with bloating, flatulence, and change in bowel habits (diarrhea or constipation) that improves with defecation; classically seen in middle-aged females

B. Related to disturbed intestinal motility; no identifiable pathologic changes

C. Increased dietary fiber may improve symptoms.

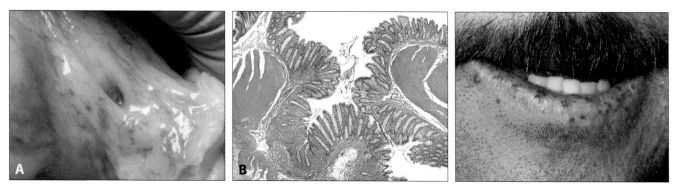

Fig. 10.23 Colonic diverticula. **A**, Gross appearance. **B**, Microscopic appearance.

Fig. 10.24 Hereditary hemorrhagic telangiectasia. (Courtesy of Drs. H. Fred and H. van Dijk, *Images of Memorable Cases*)

VII. **COLONIC POLYPS**
  A. Raised protrusions of colonic mucosa
  B. Most common types are hyperplastic and adenomatous polyps.
    1. Hyperplastic polyps are due to hyperplasia of glands; classically show a 'serrated' appearance on microscopy
      i. Most common type of polyp; usually arise in the left colon (rectosigmoid)
      ii. Benign, with no malignant potential
    2. Adenomatous polyps are due to neoplastic proliferation of glands (Fig. 10.25); 2nd most common type of colonic polyp
      i. Benign, but premalignant; may progress to adenocarcinoma via the adenoma-carcinoma sequence
    3. Adenoma-carcinoma sequence describes the molecular progression from normal colonic mucosa to adenomatous polyp to carcinoma.
      i. *APC* (adenomatous polyposis coli gene) mutations (sporadic or germline) increase risk for formation of polyp.
      ii. K-*ras* mutation leads to formation of polyp.
      iii. p53 mutation and increased expression of COX allow for progression to carcinoma; aspirin impedes progression from adenoma to carcinoma.
  C. Screening for polyps is performed by colonoscopy and testing for fecal occult blood; polyps are usually clinically silent, but can bleed.
    1. Goal is to remove adenomatous polyps before progression to carcinoma.
  D. On colonoscopy, hyperplastic and adenomatous polyps look identical. Hence, all polyps are removed and examined microscopically.
    1. Greatest risk for progression from adenoma to carcinoma is related to size > 2 cm, sessile growth, and villous histology.

VIII. **FAMILIAL ADENOMATOUS POLYPOSIS (FAP)**
  A. Autosomal dominant disorder characterized by 100s to 1000s of adenomatous colonic polyps (Fig. 10.26)
  B. Due to inherited *APC* mutation (chromosome 5); increases propensity to develop adenomatous polyps throughout colon and rectum
  C. Colon and rectum are removed prophylactically; otherwise, almost all patients develop carcinoma by 40 years of age.
  D. Gardner syndrome is FAP with fibromatosis and osteomas.
    1. Fibromatosis is a non-neoplastic proliferation of fibroblasts; arises in retroperitoneum (desmoid) and locally destroys tissue
    2. Osteoma is a benign tumor of bone that usually arises in the skull.
  E. Turcot syndrome is FAP with CNS tumors (medulloblastoma and glial tumors).

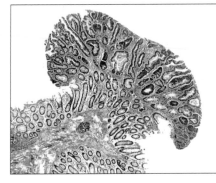

Fig. 10.25 Adenomatous polyp.

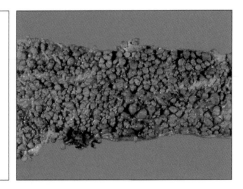

Fig. 10.26 Familial adenomatous polyposis. (Courtesy of humpath.com)

IX. JUVENILE POLYP

A. Sporadic, hamartomatous (benign) polyp that arises in children (< 5 years)
   1. Usually presents as a solitary rectal polyp that prolapses and bleeds
B. Juvenile polyposis is characterized by multiple juvenile polyps in the stomach and colon; large numbers of juvenile polyps increase the risk of progression to carcinoma.

X. PEUTZ-JEGHERS SYNDROME

A. Hamartomatous (benign) polyps throughout GI tract and mucocutaneous hyperpigmentation (freckle-like spots) on lips, oral mucosa, and genital skin; autosomal dominant disorder
B. Increased risk for colorectal, breast, and gynecologic cancer

XI. COLORECTAL CARCINOMA

A. Carcinoma arising from colonic or rectal mucosa; 3rd most common site of cancer and 3rd most common cause of cancer-related death
   1. Peak incidence is 60–70 years of age.
B. Most commonly arises from adenoma-carcinoma sequence; a second important molecular pathway is microsatellite instability (MSI).
   1. Microsatellites are repeating sequences of noncoding DNA; integrity of sequence (stability) is maintained during cell division.
   2. Instability indicates defective DNA copy mechanisms (e.g., DNA mismatch repair enzymes).
   3. Hereditary nonpolyposis colorectal carcinoma (HNPCC) is due to inherited mutations in DNA mismatch repair enzymes.
      i. Increased risk for colorectal, ovarian, and endometrial carcinoma
      ii. Colorectal carcinoma arises de novo (not from adenomatous polyps) at a relatively early age; usually right-sided
C. Screening for colorectal carcinoma occurs via colonoscopy and fecal occult blood testing; begins at 50 years of age
   1. Goal is to remove adenomatous polyps before carcinoma develops and to detect cancer early (before clinical symptoms arise).
D. Carcinoma can develop anywhere along entire length of colon.
   1. Left-sided carcinoma usually grows as a 'napkin-ring' lesion; presents with decreased stool caliber, left lower quadrant pain, and blood-streaked stool
   2. Right-sided carcinoma usually grows as a raised lesion; presents with iron-deficiency anemia (occult bleeding) and vague pain. An older adult with iron deficiency anemia has colorectal carcinoma until proven otherwise.
E. Colonic carcinoma is associated with an increased risk for *Streptococcus bovis* endocarditis.
F. Staging
   1. T—depth of invasion; tumors limited to the mucosa generally do not spread due to lack of lymphatics in the mucosa.
   2. N—spread to regional lymph nodes
   3. M—distant spread; most commonly involves the liver
G. CEA is a serum tumor marker that is useful for assessing treatment response and detecting recurrence; not useful for screening

Exocrine Pancreas, Gallbladder, and Liver Pathology

11

EXOCRINE PANCREAS

I. **ANNULAR PANCREAS**
  A. Developmental malformation in which the pancreas forms a ring around the duodenum; risk of duodenal obstruction

II. **ACUTE PANCREATITIS**
  A. Inflammation and hemorrhage of the pancreas
  B. Due to autodigestion of pancreatic parenchyma by pancreatic enzymes
      1. Premature activation of trypsin leads to activation of other pancreatic enzymes.
  C. Results in liquefactive hemorrhagic necrosis of the pancreas and fat necrosis of the peripancreatic fat (Fig. 11.1)
  D. Most commonly due to alcohol and gallstones; other causes include trauma, hypercalcemia, hyperlipidemia, drugs, scorpion stings, mumps, and rupture of a posterior duodenal ulcer.
  E. Clinical features
      1. Epigastric abdominal pain that radiates to the back
      2. Nausea and vomiting
      3. Periumbilical and flank hemorrhage (necrosis spreads into the periumbilical soft tissue and retroperitoneum)
      4. Elevated serum lipase and amylase; lipase is more specific for pancreatic damage.
      5. Hypocalcemia (calcium is consumed during saponification in fat necrosis)
  F. Complications
      1. Shock—due to peripancreatic hemorrhage and fluid sequestration
      2. Pancreatic pseudocyst—formed by fibrous tissue surrounding liquefactive necrosis and pancreatic enzymes
          i. Presents as an abdominal mass with persistently elevated serum amylase
          ii. Rupture is associated with release of enzymes into the abdominal cavity and hemorrhage.
      3. Pancreatic abscess—often due to *E coli*; presents with abdominal pain, high fever, and persistently elevated amylase
      4. DIC and ARDS

III. **CHRONIC PANCREATITIS**
  A. Fibrosis of pancreatic parenchyma, most often secondary to recurrent acute pancreatitis
      1. Most commonly due to alcohol (adults) and cystic fibrosis (children); however, many cases are idiopathic.
  B. Clinical features
      1. Epigastric abdominal pain that radiates to the back
      2. Pancreatic insufficiency—results in malabsorption with steatorrhea and fat-soluble vitamin deficiencies. Amylase and lipase are not useful serologic markers of chronic pancreatitis.
      3. Dystrophic calcification of pancreatic parenchyma on imaging; contrast studies reveal a 'chain of lakes' pattern due to dilatation of pancreatic ducts.

4. Secondary diabetes mellitus—late complication due to destruction of islets
5. Increased risk for pancreatic carcinoma

IV. **PANCREATIC CARCINOMA**
   A. Adenocarcinoma arising from the pancreatic ducts
      1. Most commonly seen in the elderly (average age is 70 years)
   B. Major risk factors are smoking and chronic pancreatitis.
   C. Clinical features (usually occur late in disease)
      1. Epigastric abdominal pain and weight loss
      2. Obstructive jaundice with pale stools and palpable gallbladder; associated with tumors that arise in the head of the pancreas (most common location)
      3. Secondary diabetes mellitus; associated with tumors that arise in the body or tail
      4. Pancreatitis
      5. Migratory thrombophlebitis (Trousseau sign); presents as swelling, erythema, and tenderness in the extremities (seen in 10% of patients)
      6. Serum tumor marker is CA 19-9.
   D. Surgical resection involves en bloc removal of the head and neck of pancreas, proximal duodenum, and gallbladder (Whipple procedure).
   E. Very poor prognosis; 1-year survival is < 10%.

GALLBLADDER AND BILIARY TRACT

I. **BILIARY ATRESIA**
   A. Failure to form or early destruction of extrahepatic biliary tree
   B. Leads to biliary obstruction within the first 2 months of life
   C. Presents with jaundice and progresses to cirrhosis

II. **CHOLELITHIASIS (GALLSTONES)**
   A. Solid, round stones in the gallbladder
   B. Due to precipitation of cholesterol (cholesterol stones) or bilirubin (bilirubin stones) in bile
      1. Arises with (1) supersaturation of cholesterol or bilirubin, (2) decreased phospholipids (e.g., lecithin) or bile acids (normally increase solubility), or (3) stasis
   C. Cholesterol stones (yellow) are the most common type (90%), especially in the West (Fig. 11.2A).
      1. Usually radiolucent (10% are radiopaque due to associated calcium)
      2. Risk factors include age (40s), estrogen (female gender, obesity, multiple pregnancies and oral contraceptives), clofibrate, Native American ethnicity, Crohn disease, and cirrhosis.

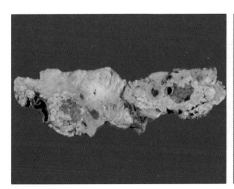

Fig. 11.1 Acute pancreatitis. (Courtesy of humpath.com)

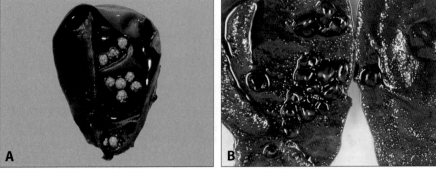

Fig. 11.2 Gallstones. **A**, Cholesterol stones. **B**, Bilirubin stones. (A, Courtesy of K.V. Santosh, MD. B, Courtesy of humpath.com)

D. Bilirubin stones (pigmented) are composed of bilirubin (Fig. 11.2B).
1. Usually radiopaque
2. Risk factors include extravascular hemolysis (increased bilirubin in bile) and biliary tract infection (e.g., *E coli, Ascaris lumbricoides,* and *Clonorchis sinensis*).
    i. *Ascaris lumbricoides* is a common roundworm that infects 25% of the world's population, especially in areas with poor sanitation (fecal-oral transmission); infects the biliary tract, increasing the risk for gallstones
    ii. *Clonorchis sinensis* is endemic in China, Korea, and Vietnam (Chinese liver fluke); infects the biliary tract, increasing the risk for gallstones, cholangitis, and cholangiocarcinoma
E. Gallstones are usually asymptomatic; complications include biliary colic, acute and chronic cholecystitis, ascending cholangitis, gallstone ileus, and gallbladder cancer.

III. BILIARY COLIC
A. Waxing and waning right upper quadrant pain
B. Due to the gallbladder contracting against a stone lodged in the cystic duct
C. Symptoms are relieved if the stone passes.
D. Common bile duct obstruction may result in acute pancreatitis or obstructive jaundice.

IV. ACUTE CHOLECYSTITIS
A. Acute inflammation of the gallbladder wall
B. Impacted stone in the cystic duct results in dilatation with pressure ischemia, bacterial overgrowth (*E coli*), and inflammation.
C. Presents with right upper quadrant pain, often radiating to right scapula, fever with ↑ WBC count, nausea, vomiting, and ↑ serum alkaline phosphatase (from duct damage)
D. Risk of rupture if left untreated

V. CHRONIC CHOLECYSTITIS
A. Chronic inflammation of the gallbladder
B. Due to chemical irritation from longstanding cholelithiasis, with or without superimposed bouts of acute cholecystitis
C. Characterized by herniation of gallbladder mucosa into the muscular wall (Rokitansky-Aschoff sinus, Fig. 11.3A)
D. Presents with vague right upper quadrant pain, especially after eating
E. Porcelain gallbladder is a late complication (Fig. 11.3B).
1. Shrunken, hard gallbladder due to chronic inflammation, fibrosis, and dystrophic calcification

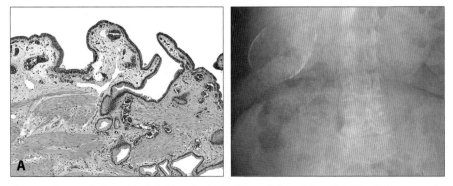

Fig. 11.3 Chronic cholecystitis. **A**, Rokitansky-Aschoff sinus. **B**, Porcelain gallbladder. (B, Courtesy of Drs. H. Fred and H. van Dijk, *Images of Memorable Cases*)

2. Increased risk for carcinoma

F. Treatment is cholecystectomy, especially if porcelain gallbladder is present.

VI. ASCENDING CHOLANGITIS

A. Bacterial infection of the bile ducts

B. Usually due to ascending infection with enteric gram-negative bacteria

C. Presents as sepsis (high fever and chills), jaundice, and abdominal pain

D. Increased incidence with choledocholithiasis (stone in biliary ducts)

VII. GALLSTONE ILEUS

A. Gallstone enters and obstructs the small bowel

B. Due to cholecystitis with fistula formation between the gallbladder and small bowel

VIII. GALLBLADDER CARCINOMA

A. Adenocarcinoma arising from the glandular epithelium that lines the gallbladder wall (Fig. 11.4)

B. Gallstones are a major risk factor, especially when complicated by porcelain gallbladder.

C. Classically presents as cholecystitis in an elderly woman

D. Poor prognosis

LIVER

I. JAUNDICE

A. Yellow discoloration of the skin (Fig. 11.5); earliest sign is scleral icterus (yellow discoloration of the sclera).

B. Due to ↑ serum bilirubin, usually > 2.5 mg/dL

C. Arises with disturbances in bilirubin metabolism (Table 11.1)

D. Normal bilirubin metabolism

1. RBCs are consumed by macrophages of the reticuloendothelial system.

2. Protoporphyrin (from heme) is converted to unconjugated bilirubin (UCB).

3. Albumin carries UCB to the liver.

4. Uridine glucuronyl transferase (UGT) in hepatocytes conjugates bilirubin.

5. Conjugated bilirubin (CB) is transferred to bile canaliculi to form bile, which is stored in the gallbladder.

6. Bile is released into the small bowel to aid in digestion.

7. Intestinal flora convert CB to urobilinogen, which is oxidized to stercobilin (makes stool brown) and urobilin (partially reabsorbed into blood and filtered by kidney, making urine yellow).

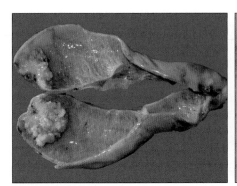

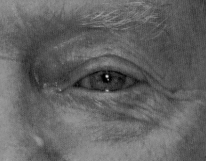

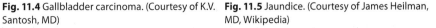

Fig. 11.4 Gallbladder carcinoma. (Courtesy of K.V. Santosh, MD)

Fig. 11.5 Jaundice. (Courtesy of James Heilman, MD, Wikipedia)

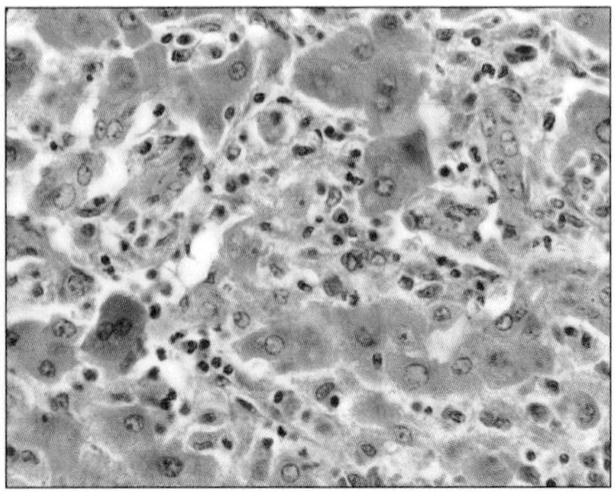

Fig. 11.6 Acute hepatitis.

Table 11.1: Causes of Jaundice

DISEASE	ETIOLOGY	LABORATORY FINDINGS	CLINICAL FEATURES
Extravascular hemolysis or Ineffective erythropoiesis	High levels of UCB overwhelm the conjugating ability of the liver.	↑ UCB	Dark urine due to ↑ urine urobilinogen (UCB is not water soluble and, thus, is absent from urine) Increased risk for pigmented bilirubin gallstones
Physiologic jaundice of the newborn	Newborn liver has transiently low UGT activity.	↑ UCB	UCB is fat soluble and can deposit in the basal ganglia (kernicterus) leading to neurological deficits and death. Treatment is phototherapy (makes UCB water soluble).
Gilbert syndrome	Mildly low UGT activity; autosomal recessive	↑ UCB	Jaundice during stress (e.g., severe infection); otherwise, not clinically significant
Crigler-Najjar syndrome	Absence of UGT	↑ UCB	Kernicterus; usually fatal
Dubin-Johnson syndrome	Deficiency of bilirubin canalicular transport protein; autosomal recessive	↑ CB	Liver is dark; otherwise, not clinically significant Rotor syndrome is similar to Dubin-Johnson syndrome, but lacks liver discoloration.
Biliary tract obstruction (obstructive jaundice)	Associated with gallstones, pancreatic carcinoma, cholangiocarcinoma, parasites, and liver fluke (*Clonorchis sinensis*)	↑ CB, ↓ urine urobilinogen, and ↑ alkaline phosphatase	Dark urine (due to bilirubinuria) and pale stool Pruritus due to ↑ plasma bile acids Hypercholesterolemia with xanthomas Steatorrhea with malabsorption of fat-soluble vitamins
Viral hepatitis	Inflammation disrupts hepatocytes and small bile ductules.	↑ in both CB and UCB	Dark urine due to ↑ urine bilirubin; urine urobilinogen is normal or decreased.

Table 11.2: Important Features of Hepatitis Viruses

VIRUS	TRANSMISSION	COMMENTS
Hepatitis A (HAV) and Hepatitis E (HEV)	Fecal-oral transmission HAV is commonly acquired by travelers. HEV is commonly acquired from contaminated water or undercooked seafood.	Acute hepatitis; no chronic state. Anti-virus IgM marks active infection. Anti-virus IgG is protective, and its presence indicates prior infection or immunization (immunization is available for HAV). HEV infection in pregnant women is associated with fulminant hepatitis (liver failure with massive liver necrosis).
Hepatitis B (HBV)	Parenteral transmission (e.g., childbirth, unprotected intercourse, intravenous drug abuse [IVDA], and needle stick)	Results in acute hepatitis; chronic disease occurs in 20% of cases (Table 11.3).
Hepatitis C (HCV)	Parenteral transmission (e.g., IVDA, unprotected intercourse); risk from transfusion is almost nonexistent due to screening of the blood supply.	Results in acute hepatitis; chronic disease occurs in most cases. HCV-RNA test confirms infection; decreased RNA levels indicate recovery; persistence indicates chronic disease.
Hepatitis D (HDV)		Dependent on HBV for infection; superinfection upon existing HBV is more severe than coinfection (infection with HBV and HDV at the same time)

Table 11.3: Serologic Markers of Hepatitis B Virus

STAGE	HBsAG	HBeAG AND HBV DNA	HBcAB	HBsAB
Acute	+ (first serologic marker to rise)	+	IgM	–
Window	–	–	IgM	–
Resolved	–	–	IgG	IgG (protective)
Chronic	+ (presence > 6 months defines chronic state)	+/–; presence of HBeAg or HBV DNA indicates infectivity.	IgG	–
Immunization	–	–	–	IgG (protective)

II. VIRAL HEPATITIS

A. Inflammation of liver parenchyma, usually due to hepatitis virus (Table 11.2); other causes include EBV and CMV.

B. Hepatitis virus causes acute hepatitis, which may progress to chronic hepatitis.

C. Acute hepatitis presents as jaundice (mixed CB and UCB) with dark urine (due to CB), fever, malaise, nausea, and elevated liver enzymes (ALT > AST).

   1. Inflammation involves lobules of the liver and portal tracts and is characterized by apoptosis of hepatocytes (Fig. 11.6).

   2. Some cases may be asymptomatic with elevated liver enzymes.

   3. Symptoms last < 6 months.

D. Chronic hepatitis is characterized by symptoms that last > 6 months.

   1. Inflammation predominantly involves portal tract (Fig. 11.7)

   2. Risk of progression to cirrhosis

III. CIRRHOSIS

A. End-stage liver damage characterized by disruption of the normal hepatic parenchyma by bands of fibrosis and regenerative nodules of hepatocytes (Fig. 11.8)

B. Fibrosis is mediated by TGF-β from stellate cells which lie beneath the endothelial cells that line the sinusoids.

C. Clinical features

   1. Portal hypertension leads to

      i. Ascites (fluid in the peritoneal cavity)

      ii. Congestive splenomegaly/hypersplenism

      iii. Portosystemic shunts (esophageal varices, hemorrhoids, and caput medusae)

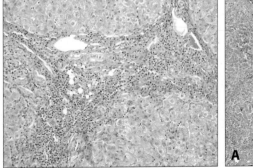

Fig. 11.7 Chronic hepatitis.

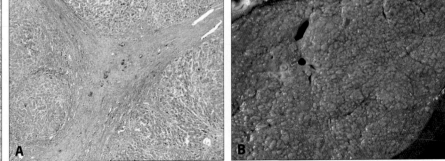

Fig. 11.8 Cirrhosis. **A**, Microscopic appearance. **B**, Gross appearance. (B, Courtesy of humpath.com)

      iv. Hepatorenal syndrome (rapidly developing renal failure secondary to cirrhosis)

   2. Decreased detoxification results in

      i. Mental status changes, asterixis, and eventual coma (due to ↑ serum ammonia); metabolic, hence reversible

      ii. Gynecomastia, spider angiomata, and palmar erythema due to hyperestrinism

      iii. Jaundice

   3. Decreased protein synthesis leads to

      i. Hypoalbuminemia with edema

      ii. Coagulopathy due to decreased synthesis of clotting factors; degree of deficiency is followed by PT.

IV. ALCOHOL-RELATED LIVER DISEASE

  A. Damage to hepatic parenchyma due to consumption of alcohol

    1. Most common cause of liver disease in the West

  B. Fatty liver is the accumulation of fat in hepatocytes (Fig. 11.9A).

    1. Results in a heavy, greasy liver; resolves with abstinence (Fig. 11.9B)

  C. Alcoholic hepatitis results from chemical injury to hepatocytes; generally seen with binge drinking

    1. Acetaldehyde (metabolite of alcohol) mediates damage.

    2. Characterized by swelling of hepatocytes with formation of Mallory bodies (damaged cytokeratin filaments, Fig. 11.10), necrosis, and acute inflammation

    3. Presents with painful hepatomegaly and elevated liver enzymes (AST > ALT); may result in death

  D. Cirrhosis is a complication of long-term, chronic alcohol-induced liver damage; occurs in 10–20% of alcoholics

V. NONALCOHOLIC FATTY LIVER DISEASE

  A. Fatty change, hepatitis, and/or cirrhosis that develop without exposure to alcohol (or other known insult)

  B. Associated with obesity

  C. Diagnosis of exclusion; ALT > AST

VI. HEMOCHROMATOSIS

  A. Excess body iron leading to deposition in tissues (hemosiderosis) and organ damage (hemochromatosis)

    1. Tissue damage is mediated by generation of free radicals.

  B. Due to autosomal recessive defect in iron absorption (primary) or chronic transfusions (secondary)

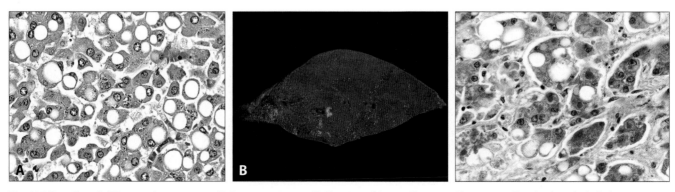

Fig. 11.9 Fatty liver. **A**, Microscopic appearance. **B**, Gross appearance. (B, Courtesy of Jerome Taxy, MD)

Fig. 11.10 Mallory bodies, alcoholic hepatitis.

1. Primary hemochromatosis is due to mutations in the *HFE* gene, usually C282Y (cysteine is replaced by tyrosine at amino acid 282).

C. Presents in late adulthood
  1. Classic triad is cirrhosis, secondary diabetes mellitus, and bronze skin; other findings include dilated cardiomyopathy, cardiac arrhythmias and gonadal dysfunction (due to testicular atrophy).
  2. Labs show ↑ ferritin, ↓ TIBC, ↑ serum iron, and ↑ % saturation.
  3. Liver biopsy reveals accumulation of brown pigment in hepatocytes (Fig. 11.11A); Prussian blue stain distinguishes iron (blue) from lipofuscin (Fig. 11.11B).
    i. Lipofuscin is a brown pigment that is a by-product from the turnover ('wear and tear') of peroxidized lipids; it is commonly present in hepatocytes (Fig. 11.11C).

D. Increased risk of hepatocellular carcinoma

E. Treatment is phlebotomy.

VII. WILSON DISEASE

A. Autosomal recessive defect (*ATP7B* gene) in ATP-mediated hepatocyte copper transport
  1. Results in lack of copper transport into bile and lack of copper incorporation into ceruloplasmin

B. Copper builds up in hepatocytes, leaks into serum, and deposits in tissues.
  1. Copper-mediated production of hydroxyl free radicals leads to tissue damage.

C. Presents in childhood with
  1. Cirrhosis
  2. Neurologic manifestations (behavioral changes, dementia, chorea, and Parkinsonian symptoms due to deposition of copper in basal ganglia)
  3. Kayser-Fleisher rings in the cornea

D. Labs show ↑ urinary copper, ↓ serum ceruloplasmin, and ↑ copper on liver biopsy.

E. Increased risk of hepatocellular carcinoma

F. Treatment is D-penicillamine (chelates copper).

VIII. PRIMARY BILIARY CIRRHOSIS

A. Autoimmune granulomatous destruction of intrahepatic bile ducts
  1. Classically arises in women (average age is 40 years)
  2. Associated with other autoimmune diseases

B. Etiology is unknown; antimitochondrial antibody is present.

C. Presents with features of obstructive jaundice

D. Cirrhosis is a late complication.

IX. PRIMARY SCLEROSING CHOLANGITIS

A. Inflammation and fibrosis of intrahepatic and extrahepatic bile ducts

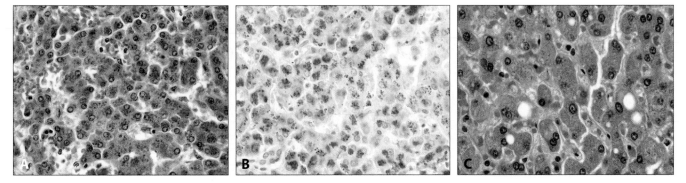

Fig. 11.11 Hemochromatosis. **A**, Iron deposition in hepatocytes. **B**, Prussian blue stain. **C**, Lipofuscin in hepatocytes for comparison.

      1. Periductal fibrosis with an 'onion-skin' appearance (Fig. 11.12)

      2. Uninvolved regions are dilated resulting in a "beaded" appearance on contrast imaging.

  B. Etiology is unknown, but associated with ulcerative colitis; p-ANCA is often positive.

  C. Presents with obstructive jaundice; cirrhosis is a late complication.

  D. Increased risk for cholangiocarcinoma

X. REYE SYNDROME

  A. Fulminant liver failure and encephalopathy in children with viral illness who take aspirin

      1. Likely related to mitochondrial damage of hepatocytes

  B. Presents with hypoglycemia, elevated liver enzymes, and nausea with vomiting; may progress to coma and death

XI. HEPATIC ADENOMA

  A. Benign tumor of hepatocytes

  B. Associated with oral contraceptive use; regresses upon cessation of drug

  C. Risk of rupture and intraperitoneal bleeding, especially during pregnancy

      1. Tumors are subcapsular and grow with exposure to estrogen.

XII. HEPATOCELLULAR CARCINOMA

  A. Malignant tumor of hepatocytes

  B. Risk factors include

      1. Chronic hepatitis (e.g., HBV and HCV)

      2. Cirrhosis (e.g., alcohol, nonalcoholic fatty liver disease, hemochromatosis, Wilson disease, and A1AT deficiency)

      3. Aflatoxins derived from *Aspergillus* (induce p53 mutations)

  C. Increased risk for Budd-Chiari syndrome

      1. Liver infarction secondary to hepatic vein obstruction

      2. Presents with painful hepatomegaly and ascites

  D. Tumors are often detected late because symptoms are masked by cirrhosis; poor prognosis

  E. Serum tumor marker is alpha-fetoprotein.

XIII. METASTASIS TO LIVER

  A. More common than primary liver tumors; most common sources include colon, pancreas, lung, and breast carcinomas.

  B. Results in multiple nodules in the liver (Fig. 11.13)

  C. Clinically may be detected as hepatomegaly with a nodular free edge of the liver

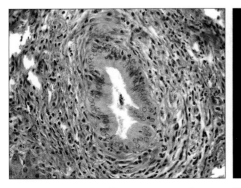

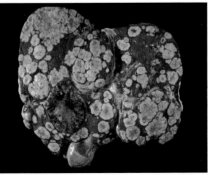

Fig. 11.12 'Onion-skin' fibrosis, primary sclerosing cholangitis.

Fig. 11.13 Metastatic carcinoma involving liver. (Courtesy of Jerome Taxy, MD)

Kidney and Urinary Tract Pathology

12

CONGENITAL

I. **HORSESHOE KIDNEY**
   A. Conjoined kidneys usually connected at the lower pole (Fig. 12.1); most common congenital renal anomaly
   B. Kidney is abnormally located in the lower abdomen; horseshoe kidney gets caught on the inferior mesenteric artery root during its ascent from the pelvis to the abdomen.

II. **RENAL AGENESIS**
   A. Absent kidney formation; may be unilateral or bilateral
   B. Unilateral agenesis leads to hypertrophy of the existing kidney; hyperfiltration increases risk of renal failure later in life.
   C. Bilateral agenesis leads to oligohydramnios with lung hypoplasia, flat face with low set ears, and developmental defects of the extremities (Potter sequence, Fig. 12.2); incompatible with life

   baby breaths amniotic fluid in to out to expand the lung

III. **DYSPLASTIC KIDNEY**
   A. Noninherited congenital malformation of the renal parenchyma characterized by cysts and abnormal tissue (e.g., cartilage, Fig. 12.3)
   B. Usually unilateral; when bilateral, must be distinguished from inherited polycystic kidney disease

IV. **POLYCYSTIC KIDNEY DISEASE (PKD)**
   A. Inherited defect leading to bilateral enlarged kidneys with cysts in the renal cortex and medulla (Fig. 12.4)
   B. Autosomal recessive form presents in infants as worsening renal failure and hypertension; newborns may present with Potter sequence.
      1. Associated with congenital hepatic fibrosis (leads to portal hypertension) and hepatic cysts
   C. Autosomal dominant form presents in young adults as hypertension (due to increased renin), hematuria, and worsening renal failure.
      1. Due to mutation in the *APKD1* or *APKD2* gene; cysts develop over time.
      2. Associated with berry aneurysm, hepatic cysts, and mitral valve prolapse
         cause death

V. **MEDULLARY CYSTIC KIDNEY DISEASE**
   A. Inherited (autosomal dominant) defect leading to cysts in the medullary collecting ducts
   B. Parenchymal fibrosis results in shrunken kidneys and worsening renal failure.

ACUTE RENAL FAILURE (ARF)

I. **BASIC PRINCIPLES**
   A. Acute, severe decrease in renal function (develops within days)
   B. Hallmark is azotemia (increased BUN and creatinine [Cr]), often with oliguria.
      ↳ ↑ Nitrogenous waste in blood

C. Divided into prerenal, postrenal, and intrarenal azotemia based on etiology

II. PRERENAL AZOTEMIA

A. Due to decreased blood flow to kidneys (e.g., cardiac failure); common cause of ARF
B. Decreased blood flow results in ↓ GFR, azotemia, and oliguria.
C. Reabsorption of fluid and BUN ensues (serum BUN:Cr ratio > 15); tubular function remains intact (fractional excretion of sodium [FENa] < 1% and urine osmolality [osm] > 500 mOsm/kg).

III. POSTRENAL AZOTEMIA

A. Due to obstruction of urinary tract downstream from the kidney (e.g., ureters)
B. Decreased outflow results in ↓ GFR, azotemia, and oliguria.
C. During early stage of obstruction, increased tubular pressure "forces" BUN into the blood (serum BUN:Cr ratio > 15); tubular function remains intact (FENa < 1% and urine osm > 500 mOsm/kg).
D. With long-standing obstruction, tubular damage ensues, resulting in decreased reabsorption of BUN (serum BUN:Cr ratio < 15), decreased reabsorption of sodium (FENa > 2%), and inability to concentrate urine (urine osm < 500 mOsm/kg).

IV. ACUTE TUBULAR NECROSIS

A. Injury and necrosis of tubular epithelial cells (Fig. 12.5); most common cause of acute renal failure (intrarenal azotemia)
B. Necrotic cells plug tubules; obstruction decreases GFR.
   1. Brown, granular casts are seen in the urine.
C. Dysfunctional tubular epithelium results in decreased reabsorption of BUN (serum BUN:Cr ratio < 15), decreased reabsorption of sodium (FENa > 2%), and inability to concentrate urine (urine osm < 500 mOsm/kg).
D. Etiology may be ischemic or nephrotoxic.
   1. Ischemia—Decreased blood supply results in necrosis of tubules.
      i. Often preceded by prerenal azotemia
      ii. Proximal tubule and medullary segment of the thick ascending limb are particularly susceptible to ischemic damage.
   2. Nephrotoxic—Toxic agents result in necrosis of tubules.
      i. Proximal tubule is particularly susceptible.
      ii. Causes include aminoglycosides (most common), heavy metals (e.g., lead), myoglobinuria (e.g., from crush injury to muscle), ethylene glycol (associated with oxalate crystals in urine), radiocontrast dye, and urate (e.g., tumor lysis syndrome).
      iii. Hydration and allopurinol are used prior to initiation of chemotherapy to decrease risk of urate-induced ATN.

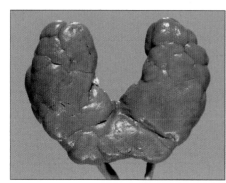

Fig. 12.1 Horseshoe kidney. (Courtesy of humpath.com)

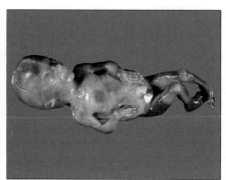

Fig. 12.2 Potter sequence. (Courtesy of humpath. com)

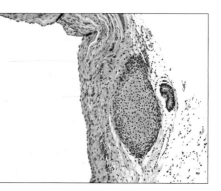

Fig. 12.3 Dysplastic kidney. (Courtesy of Aliya Husain, MD)

E. Clinical features
1. Oliguria with brown, granular casts
2. Elevated BUN and creatinine
3. Hyperkalemia (due to decreased renal excretion) with metabolic acidosis

↑ anion gap b/c you can't get rid of organic acids

F. Reversible, but often requires supportive dialysis since electrolyte imbalances can be fatal
1. Oliguria can persist for 2–3 weeks before recovery; tubular cells (stable cells) take time to reenter the cell cycle and regenerate.

V. ACUTE INTERSTITIAL NEPHRITIS
A. Drug-induced hypersensitivity involving the interstitium and tubules (Fig. 12.6); results in acute renal failure (intrarenal azotemia)
B. Causes include NSAIDs, penicillin, and diuretics.
C. Presents as oliguria, fever, and rash days to weeks after starting a drug; eosinophils may be seen in urine.
D. Resolves with cessation of drug
E. May progress to renal papillary necrosis

VI. RENAL PAPILLARY NECROSIS
A. Necrosis of renal papillae
B. Presents with gross hematuria and flank pain
C. Causes include
1. Chronic analgesic abuse (e.g., long-term phenacetin or aspirin use)
2. Diabetes mellitus
3. Sickle cell trait or disease
4. Severe acute pyelonephritis

NEPHROTIC SYNDROME

I. BASIC PRINCIPLES
A. Glomerular disorders characterized by proteinuria (> 3.5 g/day) resulting in
1. Hypoalbuminemia—pitting edema
2. Hypogammaglobulinemia—increased risk of infection
3. Hypercoagulable state—due to loss of antithrombin III
4. Hyperlipidemia and hypercholesterolemia—may result in fatty casts in urine
   (2 b/c prot)

II. MINIMAL CHANGE DISEASE (MCD)
A. Most common cause of nephrotic syndrome in children
B. Usually idiopathic; may be associated with Hodgkin lymphoma

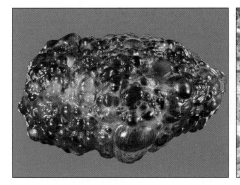
Fig. 12.4 Polycystic kidney disease. (Courtesy of Jamie Steinmetz, MD)

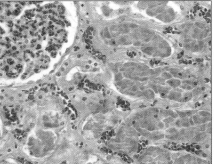
Fig. 12.5 Acute tubular necrosis.

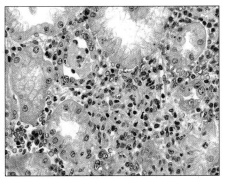
Fig. 12.6 Acute interstitial nephritis.

C. Normal glomeruli on H&E stain (Fig. 12.7A); lipid may be seen in proximal tubule cells.

D. Effacement of foot processes on electron microscopy (EM, Fig. 12.7B)

due to cytokines

E. No immune complex deposits; negative immunofluorescence (IF)

F. Selective proteinuria (loss of albumin, but not immunoglobulin)

G. Excellent response to steroids (damage is mediated by cytokines from T cells)

mesangium holds capillary loops together

III. FOCAL SEGMENTAL GLOMERULOSCLEROSIS (FSGS)

A. Most common cause of nephrotic syndrome in Hispanics and African Americans

B. Usually idiopathic; may be associated with HIV, heroin use, and sickle cell disease

C. Focal (some glomeruli) and segmental (involving only part of the glomerulus) sclerosis on H&E stain (Fig. 12.8)

D. Effacement of foot processes on EM

E. No immune complex deposits; negative IF

F. Poor response to steroids; progresses to chronic renal failure

IV. MEMBRANOUS NEPHROPATHY

A. Most common cause of nephrotic syndrome in Caucasian adults

B. Usually idiopathic; may be associated with hepatitis B or C, solid tumors, SLE, or drugs (e.g., NSAIDs and penicillamine)

Podocyte Membranous BM/Type II Type I endothelium

C. Thick glomerular basement membrane on H&E (Fig. 12.9A)

D. Due to immune complex deposition (granular IF, Fig. 12.9B); subepithelial deposits with 'spike and dome' appearance on EM (Fig. 12.9C)

→ die from renal failure
→ under podocytes

E. Poor response to steroids; progresses to chronic renal failure

→ of mesangial cell → cuts the deposits in 1/2

V. MEMBRANOPROLIFERATIVE GLOMERULONEPHRITIS

A. Thick glomerular basement membrane on H&E, often with 'tram-track' appearance

B. Due to immune complex deposition (granular IF)

C. Divided into two types based on location of deposits

1. Type I—subendothelial (Fig. 12.10); associated with HBV and HCV

2. Type II (dense deposit disease)—intramembranous; associated with C3 nephritic factor (autoantibody that stabilizes C3 convertase, leading to overactivation of complement, inflammation, and low levels of circulating C3)

Can produce nephrotic, nephritic or both

C3 convertase can't be broken down

D. Poor response to steroids; progresses to chronic renal failure

VI. DIABETES MELLITUS

A. High serum glucose leads to nonenzymatic glycosylation of the vascular basement membrane resulting in hyaline arteriolosclerosis.

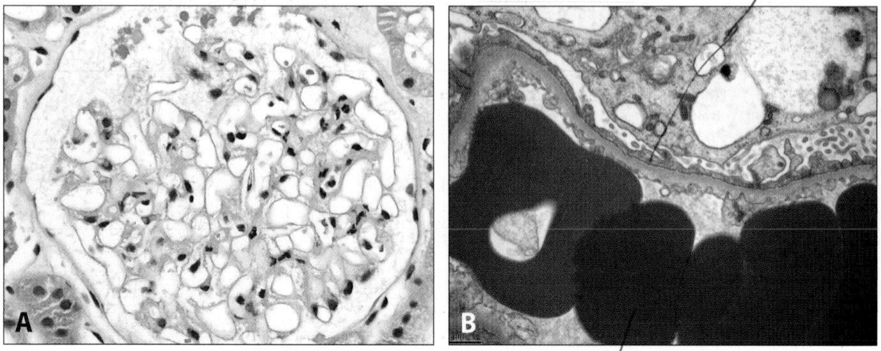

↑ thick of vessel wall = ↓ r of lumen

flat foot processes

Fig. 12.7 Minimal change disease. **A,** Normal glomerulus. **B,** Effacement of foot processes on EM. (Courtesy of Tony Chang, MD)

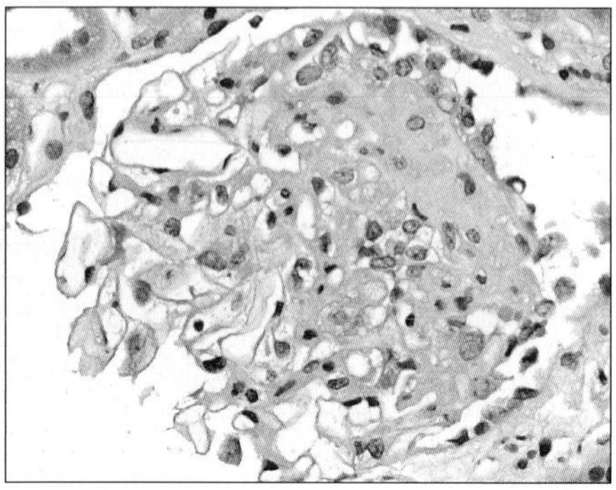

RBC

Fig. 12.8 Focal segmental glomerulosclerosis.

B. Glomerular efferent arteriole is more affected than the afferent arteriole, leading to high glomerular filtration pressure.
   1. Hyperfiltration injury leads to microalbuminuria.
C. Eventually progresses to nephrotic syndrome
   1. Characterized by sclerosis of the mesangium with formation of Kimmelstiel-Wilson nodules (Fig. 12.11)
D. ACE inhibitors slow progression of hyperfiltration-induced damage.
   b/c ANG II constricts efferent → ↑ hyperinflation

VII. SYSTEMIC AMYLOIDOSIS

A. Kidney is the most commonly involved organ in systemic amyloidosis.
B. Amyloid deposits in the mesangium, resulting in nephrotic syndrome.
C. Characterized by apple-green birefringence under polarized light after staining with Congo red

NEPHRITIC SYNDROME

I. BASIC PRINCIPLES

A. Glomerular disorders characterized by glomerular inflammation and bleeding
   1. Limited proteinuria (< 3.5 g/day)
   2. Oliguria and azotemia
   3. Salt retention with periorbital edema and hypertension
   4. RBC casts and dysmorphic RBCs in urine
B. Biopsy reveals hypercellular, inflamed glomeruli (Fig. 12.12).

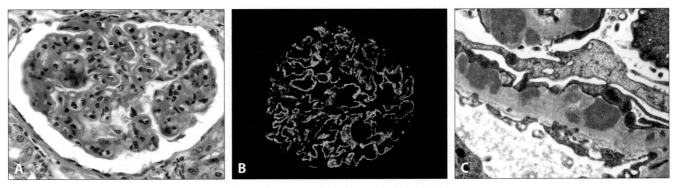

Fig. 12.9 Membranous nephropathy. **A**, Thick glomerular basement membranes. **B**, Granular IF. **C**, Subepithelial deposits with 'spike and dome' appearance. (Courtesy of Tony Chang, MD)

Kimmelstiel - Wilson nodule

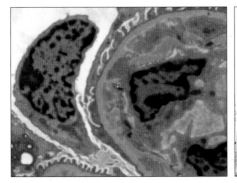

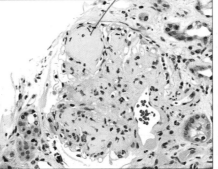

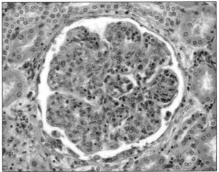

Fig. 12.10 Subendothelial deposits, membranoproliferative glomerulonephritis (type I). (Courtesy of Tony Chang, MD)

Fig. 12.11 Kimmelstiel-Wilson nodules, diabetic nephropathy.

Fig. 12.12 Hypercellular, inflamed glomerulus, nephritic syndrome.

1. Immune-complex deposition activates complement; C5a attracts neutrophils, which mediate damage.

II. POSTSTREPTOCOCCAL GLOMERULONEPHRITIS (PSGN)

A. Nephritic syndrome that arises after group A β-hemolytic streptococcal infection of the skin (impetigo) or pharynx
   1. Occurs with nephritogenic strains ~ M protein
   2. May occur after infection with nonstreptococcal organisms as well

B. Presents 2–3 weeks after infection as hematuria (cola-colored urine), oliguria, hypertension, and periorbital edema
   1. Usually seen in children, but may occur in adults

C. Hypercellular, inflamed glomeruli on H&E

D. Mediated by immune complex deposition (granular IF); subepithelial 'humps' on EM (Fig. 12.13)

E. Treatment is supportive.
   1. Children rarely (1%) progress to renal failure.
   2. Some adults (25%) develop rapidly progressive glomerulonephritis (RPGN).

III. RAPIDLY PROGRESSIVE GLOMERULONEPHRITIS

A. Nephritic syndrome that progresses to renal failure in weeks to months

Table 12.1: Immunofluorescence Findings in Rapidly Progressive Glomerulonephritis

IMMUNOFLUORESCENCE PATTERN	DISEASE	COMMENTS
Linear (anti-basement membrane antibody, Fig. 12.15)	Goodpasture syndrome	Antibody against collagen in glomerular and alveolar basement membranes; presents as hematuria and hemoptysis, classically in young, adult males
Granular (immune complex deposition)	PSGN (most common) or diffuse proliferative glomerulonephritis *most common in SLE*	Diffuse proliferative glomerulonephritis is due to diffuse antigen-antibody complex deposition, usually sub-endothelial; most common type of renal disease in SLE
Negative IF (pauci-immune)	Wegener granulomatosis, microscopic polyangiitis, and Churg-Strauss syndrome *lungs kidneys nasal pharynx*	Wegener granulomatosis is associated with c-ANCA; microscopic polyangiitis and Churg-Strauss are associated with p-ANCA. Granulomatous inflammation, eosinophilia, and asthma distinguish Churg-Strauss from microscopic polyangiitis.

P-ANCA – next to nucleus
C-ANCA – in cytosol
anti-neutrophil

Churg - Strauss
Granulomatous
Eosinophilia
Asthma

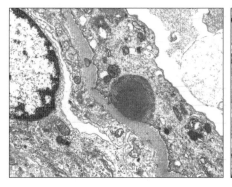

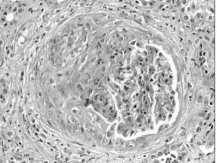

Fig. 12.13 Subepithelial 'humps,' PSGN. (Courtesy of Tony Chang, MD)

Fig. 12.14 Crescent formation, rapidly progressive glomerulonephritis.

B. Characterized by crescents in Bowman space (of glomeruli) on H&E stain; crescents are comprised of fibrin and macrophages (Fig. 12.14).

C. Clinical picture and IF help resolve etiology (Table 12.1).

IV. IgA NEPHROPATHY (BERGER DISEASE)

A. IgA immune complex deposition in mesangium of glomeruli; most common nephropathy worldwide

B. Presents during childhood as episodic gross or microscopic hematuria with RBC casts, usually following mucosal infections (e.g., gastroenteritis)

   1. IgA production is increased during infection.

C. IgA immune complex deposition in the mesangium is seen on IF (Fig. 12.16).

D. May slowly progress to renal failure

V. ALPORT SYNDROME

A. Inherited defect in type IV collagen; most commonly X-linked

B. Results in thinning and splitting of the glomerular basement membrane

C. Presents as isolated hematuria, sensory hearing loss, and ocular disturbances

URINARY TRACT INFECTION

I. BASIC PRINCIPLES

A. Infection of urethra, bladder, or kidney

B. Most commonly arises due to ascending infection; increased incidence in females

C. Risk factors include sexual intercourse, urinary stasis, and catheters.

II. CYSTITIS

A. Infection of the bladder

B. Presents as dysuria, urinary frequency, urgency, and suprapubic pain; systemic signs (e.g., fever) are usually absent.

C. Laboratory findings

   1. Urinalysis—cloudy urine with > 10 WBCs/high power field (hpf)

   2. Dipstick—Positive leukocyte esterase (due to pyuria) and nitrites (bacteria convert nitrates to nitrites)

   3. Culture—greater than 100,000 colony forming units (gold standard)

D. Etiology

   1. *E coli* (80%)

   2. *Staphylococcus saprophyticus*—increased incidence in young, sexually active women (but *E coli* is still more common in this population)

   3. *Klebsiella pneumoniae*

   4. *Proteus mirabilis*—alkaline urine with ammonia scent

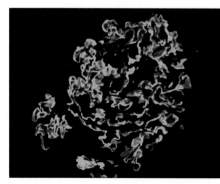

Fig. 12.15 Linear IF, Goodpasture syndrome. (Courtesy of Tony Chang, MD)

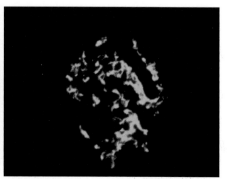

Fig. 12.16 IgA nephropathy. (Courtesy of Tony Chang, MD)

    5. *Enterococcus faecalis*

E. Sterile pyuria is the presence of pyuria (> 10 WBCs/hpf and leukocyte esterase) with a negative urine culture.

    1. Suggests urethritis due to *Chlamydia trachomatis* or *Neisseria gonorrhoeae* (dominant presenting sign of urethritis is dysuria)

III. PYELONEPHRITIS

A. Infection of the kidney

    1. Usually due to ascending infection; increased risk with vesicoureteral reflux

B. Presents with fever, flank pain, WBC casts, and leukocytosis in addition to symptoms of cystitis

C. Most common pathogens are

    1. *E coli* (90%)

    2. *Enterococcus faecalis*

    3. *Klebsiella* species

IV. CHRONIC PYELONEPHRITIS

A. Interstitial fibrosis and atrophy of tubules due to multiple bouts of acute pyelonephritis

B. Due to vesicoureteral reflux (children) or obstruction (e.g., BPH or cervical carcinoma)

C. Leads to cortical scarring with blunted calyces; scarring at upper and lower poles is characteristic of vesicoureteral reflux.

D. Atrophic tubules containing eosinophilic proteinaceous material resemble thyroid follicles ('thyroidization' of the kidney, Fig. 12.17); waxy casts may be seen in urine.

[handwritten margin note: the ♀ @ which ureter meets bladder prevents reflux]

NEPHROLITHIASIS

I. BASIC PRINCIPLES

A. Precipitation of a urinary solute as a stone (Table 12.2)

B. Risk factors include high concentration of solute in the urinary filtrate and low urine volume.

C. Presents as colicky pain with hematuria and unilateral flank tenderness

    1. Stone is usually passed within hours; if not, surgical intervention may be required.

CHRONIC RENAL FAILURE

I. BASIC PRINCIPLES

A. End-stage kidney failure

    1. May result from glomerular, tubular, inflammatory, or vascular insults

    2. Most common causes are diabetes mellitus, hypertension, and glomerular disease.

B. Clinical features

    1. Uremia—Increased nitrogenous waste products in blood (azotemia) result in nausea, anorexia, pericarditis, platelet dysfunction, encephalopathy with asterixis, and deposition of urea crystals in skin.

    2. Salt and water retention with resultant hypertension

    3. Hyperkalemia with metabolic acidosis *(anion gap)*

    4. Anemia due to decreased erythropoietin production by renal peritubular interstitial cells

5. Hypocalcemia due to decreased 1-alpha-hydroxylation of vitamin D by proximal renal tubule cells and hyperphosphatemia
6. Renal osteodystrophy due to secondary hyperparathyroidism, osteomalacia, and osteoporosis ⌐osteitis fibrosa cystica⌐
C. Treatment involves dialysis or renal transplant.
    1. Cysts often develop within shrunken end-stage kidneys during dialysis, increasing risk for renal cell carcinoma.

RENAL NEOPLASIA

I. **ANGIOMYOLIPOMA**
   A. Hamartoma comprised of blood vessels, smooth muscle, and adipose tissue
   B. Increased frequency in tuberous sclerosis

II. **RENAL CELL CARCINOMA**
   A. Malignant epithelial tumor arising from kidney tubules

Table 12.2: Features of Nephrolithiasis

COMPOSITION	FREQUENCY	CAUSES	TREATMENT
Calcium oxalate and/ or calcium phosphate	Most common type; usually seen in adults	Most common cause is idiopathic hypercalciuria; hypercalcemia and its related causes must be excluded. Also seen with Crohn disease ⌐Ca²⁺ oxalate	Treatment is hydrochlorothiazide (calcium-sparing diuretic). (↓ amt of Ca in urine)
Ammonium magnesium phosphate	Second most common type	Most common cause is infection with urease-positive organisms (e.g., *Proteus vulgaris* or *Klebsiella*); alkaline urine leads to formation of stone.	Classically, results in staghorn calculi in renal calyces (Fig. 12.18), which act as a nidus for urinary tract infections. Treatment involves surgical removal of stone (due to size) and eradication of pathogen (to prevent recurrence).
Uric acid	Third most common stone (5%); radiolucent (as opposed to other types of stones which are radiopaque)	Risk factors include hot, arid climates, low urine volume, and acidic pH. Most common stone seen in patients with gout; hyperuricemia (e.g., in leukemia or myeloproliferative disorders) increases risk.	Treatment involves hydration and alkalinization of urine (potassium bicarbonate); allopurinol is also administered in patients with gout.
Cysteine	Rare cause of nephrolithiasis; most commonly seen in children	Associated with cystinuria (a genetic defect of tubules that results in decreased reabsorption of cysteine)	May form staghorn calculi; treatment involves hydration and alkalinization of urine.

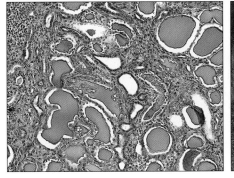

Fig. 12.17 'Thyroidization' of kidney, chronic pyelonephritis.

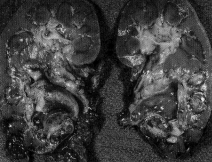

Fig. 12.18 Ammonium magnesium phosphate stone. (Courtesy of webpathology.com)

B. Presents with classic triad of hematuria, palpable mass, and flank pain
1. All three symptoms rarely occur together; hematuria is the most common symptom.
2. Fever, weight loss, or paraneoplastic syndrome (e.g., EPO, renin, PTHrP, or ACTH) may also be present.
3. Rarely may present with left-sided varicocele
    i. Involvement of the left renal vein by carcinoma blocks drainage of the left spermatic vein leading to varicocele.
    ii. Right spermatic vein drains directly into the IVC; hence, right-sided varicocele is not seen.
C. Gross exam reveals a yellow mass (Fig. 12.19A); microscopically, the most common variant exhibits clear cytoplasm (clear cell type, Fig. 12.19B).
D. Pathogenesis involves loss of *VHL* (3p) tumor suppressor gene, which leads to increased IGF-1 (promotes growth) and increased HIF transcription factor (increases VEGF and PDGF).
E. Tumors may be hereditary or sporadic.
1. Sporadic tumors classically arise in adult males (average age is 60 years) as a single tumor in the upper pole of the kidney; major risk factor for sporadic tumors is cigarette smoke.
2. Hereditary tumors arise in younger adults and are often bilateral.
    i. Von Hippel-Lindau disease is an autosomal dominant disorder associated with inactivation of the *VHL* gene leading to increased risk for hemangioblastoma of the cerebellum and renal cell carcinoma.
F. Staging
1. T—based on size and involvement of the renal vein (occurs commonly and increases risk of hematogenous spread to the lungs and bone)
2. N—spread to retroperitoneal lymph nodes

III. **WILMS TUMOR**
A. Malignant kidney tumor comprised of blastema (immature kidney mesenchyme), primitive glomeruli and tubules, and stromal cells (Fig. 12.20)
1. Most common malignant renal tumor in children; average age is 3 years.
B. Presents as a large, unilateral flank mass with hematuria and hypertension (due to renin secretion)
C. Most cases (90%) are sporadic; syndromic tumors may be seen with
1. WAGR syndrome—**W**ilms tumor, **A**niridia, **G**enital abnormalities, and mental and motor **R**etardation; associated with *deletion of WT1* tumor suppressor gene (located at 11p13)
2. Denys-Drash syndrome—Wilms tumor, progressive renal (glomerular) disease, and male pseudohermaphroditism; associated with *mutations of WT1*

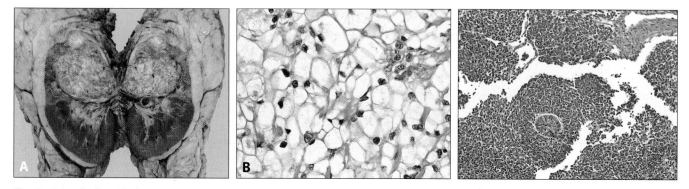

Fig. 12.19 Renal cell carcinoma. **A**, Gross appearance. **B**, Microscopic appearance.   **Fig. 12.20** Wilms tumor.

3. Beckwith-Wiedemann syndrome—Wilms tumor, neonatal hypoglycemia, muscular hemihypertrophy, and organomegaly (including tongue); associated with mutations in *WT2* gene cluster (imprinted genes at 11p15.5), particularly IGF-2

LOWER URINARY TRACT CARCINOMA

I. **UROTHELIAL (TRANSITIONAL CELL) CARCINOMA**
   A. Malignant tumor arising from the urothelial lining of the renal pelvis, ureter, bladder, or urethra
      1. Most common type of lower urinary tract cancer; usually arises in the bladder
   B. Major risk factor is cigarette smoke; additional risk factors are naphthylamine, azo dyes, and long-term cyclophosphamide or phenacetin use.
   C. Generally seen in older adults; classically presents with painless hematuria
   D. Arises via two distinct pathways (Fig. 12.21)
      1. Flat—develops as a high-grade flat tumor and then invades; associated with early p53 mutations
      2. Papillary—develops as a low-grade papillary tumor that progresses to a high-grade papillary tumor and then invades; not associated with early p53 mutations
   E. Tumors are often multifocal and recur ("field defect").

II. **SQUAMOUS CELL CARCINOMA**
   A. Malignant proliferation of squamous cells, usually involving the bladder
   B. Arises in a background of squamous metaplasia (normal bladder surface is not lined by squamous epithelium)
   C. Risk factors include chronic cystitis (older woman), *Schistosoma hematobium* infection (Egyptian male), and long-standing nephrolithiasis.

III. **ADENOCARCINOMA**
   A. Malignant proliferation of glands, usually involving bladder
   B. Arises from a urachal remnant (tumor develops at the dome of the bladder), cystitis glandularis, or exstrophy (congenital failure to form the caudal portion of the anterior abdominal and bladder walls)

[handwritten margin notes: urachus bladder — yolk sac; columnar metaplasia in response to chronic inflammation]

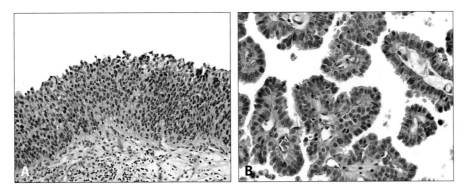

Fig. 12.21 Urothelial carcinoma. **A**, Flat. **B**, Papillary.

Female Genital System and Gestational Pathology

13

VULVA

I. **BASIC PRINCIPLES**
  A. Anatomically includes the skin and mucosa of the female genitalia external to the hymen (labia majora, labia minora, mons pubis, and vestibule)
  B. Lined by squamous epithelium

II. **BARTHOLIN CYST**
  A. Cystic dilation of the Bartholin gland
    1. One Bartholin gland is present on each side of the vaginal canal and produces mucus-like fluid that drains via ducts into the lower vestibule.
  B. Arises due to inflammation and obstruction of gland
    1. Usually occurs in women of reproductive age
  C. Presents as a unilateral, painful cystic lesion at the lower vestibule adjacent to the vaginal canal

III. **CONDYLOMA**
  A. Warty neoplasm of vulvar skin, often large
  B. Most commonly due to HPV types 6 or 11 (condyloma acuminatum, Fig. 13.1A); secondary syphilis (condyloma latum) is a less common cause. Both are sexually transmitted.
  C. Histologically, HPV-associated condylomas are characterized by koilocytes (hallmark of HPV-infected cells, Fig. 13.1B).
  D. Condylomas rarely progress to carcinoma (6 and 11 are low-risk HPV types).

IV. **LICHEN SCLEROSIS**
  A. Characterized by thinning of the epidermis and fibrosis (sclerosis) of the dermis
  B. Presents as a white patch (leukoplakia) with parchment-like vulvar skin
  C. Most commonly seen in postmenopausal women; possible autoimmune etiology
  D. Benign, but associated with a slightly increased risk for squamous cell carcinoma

V. **LICHEN SIMPLEX CHRONICUS**
  A. Characterized by hyperplasia of the vulvar squamous epithelium
  B. Presents as leukoplakia with thick, leathery vulvar skin
  C. Associated with chronic irritation and scratching
  D. Benign; no increased risk of squamous cell carcinoma

VI. **VULVAR CARCINOMA**
  A. Carcinoma arising from squamous epithelium lining the vulva
  B. Relatively rare, accounting for only a small percentage of female genital cancers
  C. Presents as leukoplakia; biopsy may be required to distinguish carcinoma from other causes of leukoplakia.
  D. Etiology may be HPV-related or non-HPV related.
  E. HPV-related vulvar carcinoma is due to high-risk HPV types 16 and 18.

1. Risk factors are related to HPV exposure and include multiple partners and early first age of intercourse; generally occurs in women of reproductive age
2. Arises from vulvar intraepithelial neoplasia (VIN), a dysplastic precursor lesion characterized by koilocytic change, disordered cellular maturation, nuclear atypia, and increased mitotic activity

F. Non-HPV related vulvar carcinoma arises, most often, from long-standing lichen sclerosis.
  1. Chronic inflammation and irritation eventually lead to carcinoma.
  2. Generally seen in elderly women (average age is > 70 years)

VII. **EXTRAMAMMARY PAGET DISEASE**
  A. Characterized by malignant epithelial cells in the epidermis of the vulva (Fig. 13.2)
  B. Presents as erythematous, pruritic, ulcerated vulvar skin
  C. Represents carcinoma in situ, usually with no underlying carcinoma
    1. Paget disease of the nipple is also characterized by malignant epithelial cells in the epidermis of the nipple, but it is almost always associated with an underlying carcinoma.
  D. Must be distinguished from melanoma, which rarely can occur on the vulva
    1. Paget cells are PAS+, keratin+, and S100-.
    2. Melanoma is PAS-, keratin-, and S100+.

VAGINA

I. **BASIC PRINCIPLES**
  A. Canal leading to the cervix
  B. Mucosa is lined by non-keratinizing squamous epithelium

II. **ADENOSIS**
  A. Focal persistence of columnar epithelium in the upper vagina
    1. During development, squamous epithelium from the lower 1/3 of the vagina (derived from the urogenital sinus) grows upward to replace the columnar epithelium lining of the upper 2/3 of the vagina (derived from the Müllerian ducts).
  B. Increased incidence in females who were exposed to diethylstilbestrol (DES) in utero

III. **CLEAR CELL ADENOCARCINOMA**
  A. Malignant proliferation of glands with clear cytoplasm
  B. Rare, but feared, complication of DES-associated vaginal adenosis

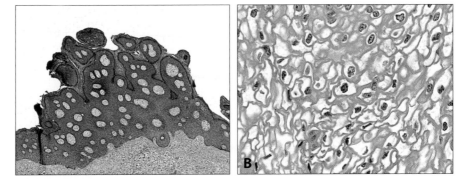

Fig. 13.1 Condyloma acuminata. **A,** Microscopic appearance. **B,** Koilocytic change.

C. Discovery of this complication (along with other DES-induced abnormalities of the gynecologic tract such as abnormal shape of the uterus) led to cessation of DES usage.

IV. EMBRYONAL RHABDOMYOSARCOMA

A. Malignant mesenchymal proliferation of immature skeletal muscle; rare

B. Presents as bleeding and a grape-like mass protruding from the vagina or penis of a child (usually < 5 yrs of age); also known as sarcoma botryoides (Fig. 13.3)

C. Rhabdomyoblast, the characteristic cell, exhibits cytoplasmic cross-striations and positive immunohistochemical staining for desmin and myogenin.

V. VAGINAL CARCINOMA

A. Carcinoma arising from squamous epithelium lining the vaginal mucosa

B. Usually related to high-risk HPV

C. Precursor lesion is vaginal intraepithelial neoplasia (VAIN).

D. When spread to regional lymph nodes occurs, cancer from the lower 1/3 of vagina goes to inguinal nodes, and cancer from the upper 2/3 goes to regional iliac nodes.

CERVIX

I. BASIC PRINCIPLES

A. Anatomically, comprises the "neck" of the uterus

B. Divided into the exocervix (visible on vaginal exam) and endocervix

  1. Exocervix is lined by nonkeratinizing squamous epithelium.

  2. Endocervix is lined by a single layer of columnar cells.

  3. Junction between the exocervix and endocervix is called the transformation zone (Fig. 13.4A).

II. HPV

A. Sexually transmitted DNA virus that infects the lower genital tract, especially the cervix in the transformation zone

B. Infection is usually eradicated by acute inflammation; persistent infection leads to an increased risk for cervical dysplasia (cervical intraepithelial neoplasia, CIN).

C. Risk of CIN depends on HPV type, which is determined by DNA sequencing.

  1. High-risk—HPV types 16, 18, 31, and 33

  2. Low-risk—HPV types 6 and 11

D. High-risk HPV produce E6 and E7 proteins which result in increased destruction of p53 and Rb, respectively. Loss of these tumor suppressor proteins increases the risk for CIN.

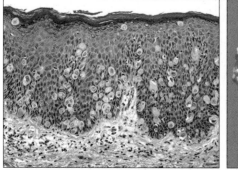

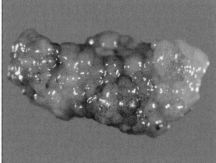

Fig. 13.2 Extramammary Paget disease of the vulva. (Courtesy of webpathology.com)

Fig. 13.3 Embryonal rhabdomyosarcoma. (Courtesy of humpath.com)

III. **CERVICAL INTRAEPITHELIAL NEOPLASIA**
   A. Characterized by koilocytic change, disordered cellular maturation, nuclear atypia, and increased mitotic activity within the cervical epithelium.
   B. Divided into grades based on the extent of epithelial involvement by immature dysplastic cells
      1. CIN I involves < 1/3 of the thickness of the epithelium.
      2. CIN II involves < 2/3 of the thickness of the epithelium.
      3. CIN III involves slightly less than the entire thickness of the epithelium (Fig. 13.4B).
      4. Carcinoma in situ (CIS) involves the entire thickness of the epithelium.
   C. CIN classically progresses in a stepwise fashion through CIN I, CIN II, CIN III, and CIS to become invasive squamous cell carcinoma.
      1. Progression is not inevitable (e.g., CIN I often regresses).
      2. The higher the grade of dysplasia, the more likely it is to progress to carcinoma and the less likely it is to regress to normal.

IV. **CERVICAL CARCINOMA**
   A. Invasive carcinoma that arises from the cervical epithelium
   B. Most commonly seen in middle-aged women (average age is 40–50 years)
   C. Presents as vaginal bleeding, especially postcoital bleeding, or cervical discharge
   D. Key risk factor is high-risk HPV infection; secondary risk factors include smoking and immunodeficiency (e.g., cervical carcinoma is an AIDS-defining illness).
   E. Most common subtypes of cervical carcinoma are squamous cell carcinoma (80% of cases) and adenocarcinoma (15% of cases). Both types are related to HPV infection.
   F. Advanced tumors often invade through the anterior uterine wall into the bladder, blocking the ureters. Hydronephrosis with postrenal failure is a common cause of death in advanced cervical carcinoma.

V. **SCREENING AND PREVENTION OF CERVICAL CARCINOMA**
   A. The goal of screening is to catch dysplasia (CIN) before it develops into carcinoma.
      1. Progression from CIN to carcinoma, on average, takes 10–20 years.
      2. Screening begins at age 21 and is initially performed yearly.
   B. Pap smear is the gold standard for screening.
      1. Cells are scraped from the transformation zone using a brush and analyzed under a microscope.
      2. Dysplastic cells are classified as low grade (CIN I) or high grade (CIN II and III).
      3. High-grade dysplasia is characterized by cells with hyperchromatic (dark) nuclei and high nuclear to cytoplasmic ratios (Fig. 13.4C).
   C. Pap smear is the most successful screening test developed to date.

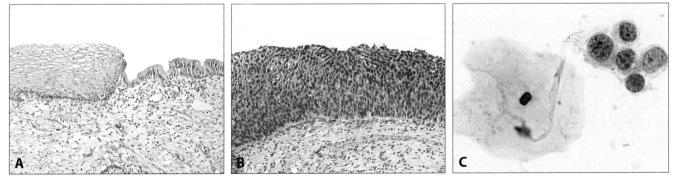

Fig. 13.4 Cervix. **A**, Cervical transformation zone, normal. **B**, CIN III. **C**, High-grade dysplasia, Pap smear. (Courtesy of Ed Uthman, MD)

1. It is responsible for a significant reduction in the morbidity and mortality of cervical carcinoma (cervical carcinoma went from being the most common to one of the least common types of gynecologic carcinoma in the US).
   2. Women who develop invasive cervical carcinoma usually have not undergone screening.
D. An abnormal Pap smear is followed by confirmatory colposcopy (visualization of cervix with a magnifying glass) and biopsy.
E. Limitations of the Pap smear include inadequate sampling of the transformation zone (false negative screening) and limited efficacy in screening for adenocarcinoma.
   1. Despite Pap smear screening, the incidence of adenocarcinoma has not decreased significantly.
F. Immunization is effective in preventing HPV infections.
   1. The quadrivalent vaccine covers HPV types 6, 11, 16, and 18.
   2. Antibodies generated against types 6 and 11 protect against condylomas.
   3. Antibodies generated against types 16 and 18 protect against CIN and carcinoma.
   4. Protection lasts for 5 years.
   5. Pap smears are still necessary due to the limited number of HPV types covered by the vaccine.

ENDOMETRIUM AND MYOMETRIUM

I. **BASIC PRINCIPLES**
   A. Endometrium is the mucosal lining of the uterine cavity.
   B. Myometrium is the smooth muscle wall underlying the endometrium (Fig. 13.5).
   C. Endometrium is hormonally sensitive.
      1. Growth of the endometrium is estrogen driven (proliferative phase).
      2. Preparation of the endometrium for implantation is progesterone driven (secretory phase).
      3. Shedding occurs with loss of progesterone support (menstrual phase).

II. **ASHERMAN SYNDROME**
   A. Secondary amenorrhea due to loss of the basalis and scarring
   B. Result of overaggressive dilation and curettage (D&C)

III. **ANOVULATORY CYCLE**
   A. Lack of ovulation
   B. Results in an estrogen-driven proliferative phase without a subsequent progesterone-driven secretory phase
      1. Proliferative glands break down and shed resulting in uterine bleeding.

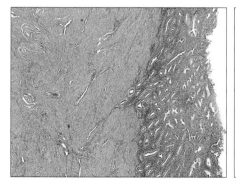

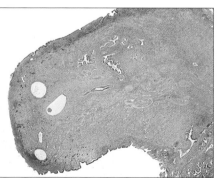

Fig. 13.5 Endometrium overlying myometrium, normal.

Fig. 13.6 Endometrial polyp.

2. Represents a common cause of dysfunctional uterine bleeding, especially during menarche and menopause

IV. **ACUTE ENDOMETRITIS**
A. Bacterial infection of the endometrium
B. Usually due to retained products of conception (e.g., after delivery or miscarriage); retained products act as a nidus for infection.
C. Presents as fever, abnormal uterine bleeding, and pelvic pain

V. **CHRONIC ENDOMETRITIS**
A. Chronic inflammation of the endometrium
B. Characterized by lymphocytes and plasma cells
1. Plasma cells are necessary for the diagnosis of chronic endometritis given that lymphocytes are normally found in the endometrium.
C. Causes include retained products of conception, chronic pelvic inflammatory disease (e.g., *Chlamydia*), IUD, and TB.
D. Presents as abnormal uterine bleeding, pain, and infertility

VI. **ENDOMETRIAL POLYP**
A. Hyperplastic protrusion of endometrium (Fig. 13.6)
B. Presents as abnormal uterine bleeding
C. Can arise as a side effect of tamoxifen, which has anti-estrogenic effects on the breast but weak pro-estrogenic effects on the endometrium

VII. **ENDOMETRIOSIS**
A. Endometrial glands and stroma outside of the uterine endometrial lining
1. Most likely due to retrograde menstruation with implantation at an ectopic site
B. Presents as dysmenorrhea (pain during menstruation) and pelvic pain; may cause infertility
1. Endometriosis cycles just like normal endometrium.
C. Most common site of involvement is the ovary, which classically results in formation of a 'chocolate' cyst (Fig. 13.7A).
1. Other sites of involvement include the uterine ligaments (pelvic pain), pouch of Douglas (pain with defecation), bladder wall (pain with urination), bowel serosa (abdominal pain and adhesions), and fallopian tube mucosa (scarring increases risk for ectopic tubal pregnancy); implants classically appear as yellow-brown 'gun-powder' nodules (Fig. 13.7B).
2. Involvement of the uterine myometrium is called adenomyosis.
D. There is an increased risk of carcinoma at the site of endometriosis, especially in the ovary.

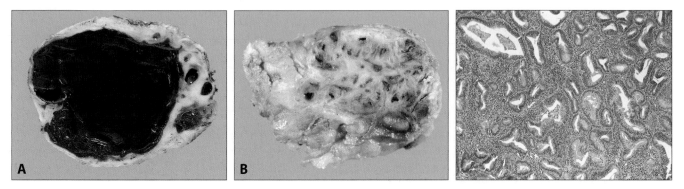

Fig. 13.7 Endometriosis. **A**, 'Chocolate cyst' of ovary. **B**, 'Gun powder' nodules. (A, Courtesy of Bulent Celasun, MD. B, Courtesy of humpath.com)   **Fig. 13.8** Endometrial hyperplasia. (Courtesy of Ed Uthman, MD)

VIII. **ENDOMETRIAL HYPERPLASIA**

A. Hyperplasia of endometrial glands relative to stroma (Fig. 13.8)

B. Occurs as a consequence of unopposed estrogen (e.g., obesity, polycystic ovary syndrome, and estrogen replacement)

C. Classically presents as postmenopausal uterine bleeding

D. Classified histologically based on architectural growth pattern (simple or complex) and the presence or absence of cellular atypia

1. Most important predictor for progression to carcinoma (major complication) is the presence of cellular atypia; simple hyperplasia with atypia often progresses to cancer (30%); whereas, complex hyperplasia without atypia rarely does (<5%).

IX. **ENDOMETRIAL CARCINOMA**

A. Malignant proliferation of endometrial glands (Fig. 13.9A)

1. Most common invasive carcinoma of the female genital tract

B. Presents as postmenopausal bleeding

C. Arises via two distinct pathways: hyperplasia and sporadic

D. In the hyperplasia pathway (75% of cases), carcinoma arises from endometrial hyperplasia.

1. Risk factors are related to estrogen exposure and include early menarche/late menopause, nulliparity, infertility with anovulatory cycles, and obesity.

2. Average age of presentation is 60 years.

3. Histology is endometrioid (i.e., normal endometrium-like, Fig. 13.9B).

E. In the sporadic pathway (25% of cases), carcinoma arises in an atrophic endometrium with no evident precursor lesion.

1. Average age at presentation is 70 years.

2. Histology is usually serous and is characterized by papillary structures (Fig. 13.9C) with psammoma body formation; p53 mutation is common, and the tumor exhibits aggressive behavior.

X. **LEIOMYOMA (FIBROIDS)**

A. Benign neoplastic proliferation of smooth muscle arising from myometrium; most common tumor in females

B. Related to estrogen exposure

1. Common in premenopausal women

2. Often multiple

3. Enlarge during pregnancy; shrink after menopause

C. Gross exam shows multiple, well-defined, white, whorled masses that may distort the uterus and impinge on pelvic structures (Fig. 13.10).

D. Usually asymptomatic; when present, symptoms include abnormal uterine bleeding, infertility, and a pelvic mass.

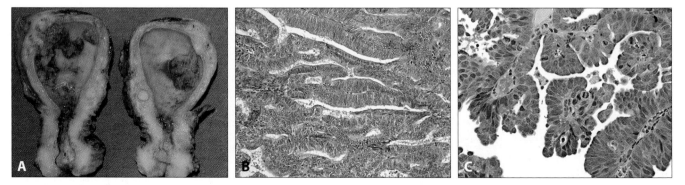

Fig. 13.9 Endometrial carcinoma. **A**, Gross appearance. **B**, Endometrioid type. **C**, Serous type. (A, Courtesy of www.anatomiapatologica.com.br)

XI. **LEIOMYOSARCOMA**
A. Malignant proliferation of smooth muscle arising from the myometrium
B. Arises de novo; leiomyosarcomas do not arise from leiomyomas.
C. Usually seen in postmenopausal women
D. Gross exam often shows a single lesion with areas of necrosis and hemorrhage; histological features include necrosis, mitotic activity, and cellular atypia.

OVARY

I. **BASIC PRINCIPLES**
A. The functional unit of the ovary is the follicle.
B. A follicle consists of an oocyte surrounded by granulosa and theca cells (Fig. 13.11A)
   1. LH acts on theca cells to induce androgen production.
   2. FSH stimulates granulosa cells to convert androgen to estradiol (drives the proliferative phase of the endometrial cycle).
   3. Estradiol surge induces an LH surge, which leads to ovulation (marking the beginning of the secretory phase of the endometrial cycle).
C. After ovulation, the residual follicle becomes a corpus luteum (Fig. 13.11B), which primarily secretes progesterone (drives the secretory phase which prepares the endometrium for a possible pregnancy).
   1. Hemorrhage into a corpus luteum can result in a hemorrhagic corpus luteal cyst, especially during early pregnancy.
D. Degeneration of follicles results in follicular cysts. Small numbers of follicular cysts are common in women and have no clinical significance.

II. **POLYCYSTIC OVARIAN DISEASE (PCOD)**
A. Multiple ovarian follicular cysts due to hormone imbalance
   1. Affects roughly 5% of women of reproductive age
B. Characterized by increased LH and low FSH (LH:FSH > 2)
   1. Increased LH induces excess androgen production (from theca cells) resulting in hirsutism (excess hair in a male distribution).
   2. Androgen is converted to estrone in adipose tissue.
      i. Estrone feedback decreases FSH resulting in cystic degeneration of follicles.
      ii. High levels of circulating estrone increase risk for endometrial carcinoma.
C. Classic presentation is an obese young woman with infertility, oligomenorrhea, and hirsutism; some patients have insulin resistance and may develop type 2 diabetes mellitus 10–15 years later.

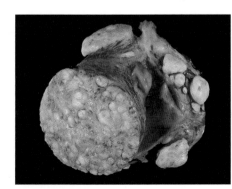

Fig. 13.10 Uterine leiomyomas. (Courtesy of Jamie Steinmetz, MD)

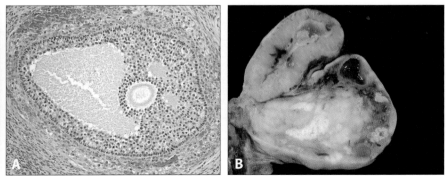

Fig. 13.11 Ovarian follicle. **A**, Normal. **B**, Corpus luteum. (B, Courtesy of Ed Uthman, MD)

OVARIAN TUMORS

I. **BASIC PRINCIPLES**
A. Ovary is composed of three cell types: surface epithelium, germ cells, and sex cord-stroma.
B. Tumor can arise from any of these cell types or from metastases.

II. **SURFACE EPITHELIAL TUMORS**
A. Most common type of ovarian tumor (70% of cases)
B. Derived from coelomic epithelium that lines the ovary; coelomic epithelium embryologically produces the epithelial lining of the fallopian tube (serous cells), endometrium, and endocervix (mucinous cells).
C. The two most common subtypes of surface epithelial tumors are serous and mucinous; both are usually cystic.
   1. Serous tumors are full of watery fluid.
   2. Mucinous tumors are full of mucus-like fluid.
D. Mucinous and serous tumors can be benign, borderline, or malignant.
   1. Benign tumors (cystadenomas) are composed of a single cyst with a simple, flat lining (Fig. 13.12); most commonly arise in premenopausal women (30–40 years old)
   2. Malignant tumors (cystadenocarcinomas) are composed of complex cysts with a thick, shaggy lining; most commonly arise in postmenopausal women (60–70 years old)
   3. Borderline tumors have features in between benign and malignant tumors.
      i. Better prognosis than clearly malignant tumors, but still carry metastatic potential
   4. *BRCA1* mutation carriers have an increased risk for serous carcinoma of the ovary and fallopian tube.
      i. *BRCA1* carriers often elect to have a prophylactic salpingo-oophorectomy (along with prophylactic mastectomy due to the increased risk for breast cancer).
E. Less common subtypes of surface epithelial tumors include endometrioid and Brenner tumor.
   1. Endometrioid tumors are composed of endometrial-like glands and are usually malignant.
      i. May arise from endometriosis
      ii. 15% of endometrioid carcinomas of the ovary are associated with an independent endometrial carcinoma (endometrioid type).
   2. Brenner tumors are composed of bladder-like epithelium and are usually benign.
F. Surface tumors clinically present late with vague abdominal symptoms (pain and fullness) or signs of compression (urinary frequency).

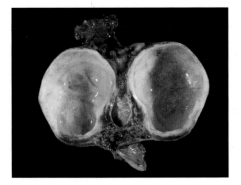

Fig. 13.12 Ovarian cystadenoma.

1. Prognosis is generally poor for surface epithelial carcinoma (worst prognosis of female genital tract cancers).
2. Epithelial carcinomas tend to spread locally, especially to the peritoneum.

G. CA-125 is a useful serum marker to monitor treatment response and screen for recurrence.

III. **GERM CELL TUMORS**

A. 2nd most common type of ovarian tumor (15% of cases)

B. Usually occur in women of reproductive age

C. Tumor subtypes mimic tissues normally produced by germ cells.
   1. Fetal tissue—cystic teratoma and embryonal carcinoma
   2. Oocytes—dysgerminoma
   3. Yolk sac—endodermal sinus tumor
   4. Placental tissue—choriocarcinoma

D. Cystic teratoma
   1. Cystic tumor composed of fetal tissue derived from two or three embryologic layers (e.g., skin, hair, bone, cartilage, gut, and thyroid, Fig. 13.13)
      i. Most common germ cell tumor in females; bilateral in 10% of cases
   2. Benign, but presence of immature tissue (usually neural) or somatic malignancy (usually squamous cell carcinoma of skin) indicates malignant potential.
   3. Struma ovarii is a teratoma composed primarily of thyroid tissue.

E. Dysgerminoma
   1. Tumor composed of large cells with clear cytoplasm and central nuclei (resemble oocytes, Fig. 13.14); most common malignant germ cell tumor
   2. Testicular counterpart is called seminoma, which is a relatively common germ cell tumor in males.
   3. Good prognosis; responds to radiotherapy
   4. Serum LDH may be elevated.

F. Endodermal sinus tumor
   1. Malignant tumor that mimics the yolk sac; most common germ cell tumor in children
   2. Serum AFP is often elevated.
   3. Schiller-Duval bodies (glomerulus-like structures) are classically seen on histology (Fig. 13.15).

G. Choriocarcinoma
   1. Malignant tumor composed of cytotrophoblasts and syncytiotrophoblasts; mimics placental tissue, but villi are absent
   2. Small, hemorrhagic tumor with early hematogenous spread
   3. High β-hCG is characteristic (produced by syncytiotrophoblasts); may lead to thecal cysts in the ovary

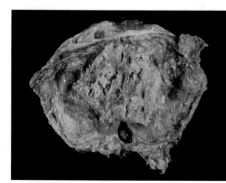

Fig. 13.13 Cystic teratoma.

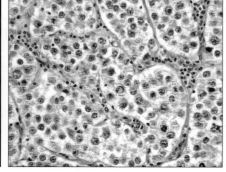

Fig. 13.14 Dysgerminoma.

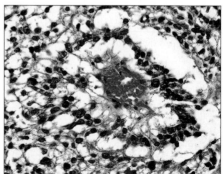

Fig. 13.15 Schiller-Duval body. (Courtesy webpathology.com)

4. Poor response to chemotherapy
H. Embryonal carcinoma
   1. Malignant tumor composed of large primitive cells
   2. Aggressive with early metastasis

IV. **SEX CORD-STROMAL TUMORS**
   A. Tumors that resemble sex cord-stromal tissues of the ovary
   B. Granulosa-theca cell tumor
      1. Neoplastic proliferation of granulosa and theca cells
      2. Often produces estrogen; presents with signs of estrogen excess
         i. Prior to puberty—precocious puberty
         ii. Reproductive age—menorrhagia or metrorrhagia
         iii. Postmenopause (most common setting for granulosa-theca cell tumors)—endometrial hyperplasia with postmenopausal uterine bleeding
      3. Malignant, but minimal risk for metastasis
   C. Sertoli-Leydig cell tumor
      1. Composed of Sertoli cells that form tubules and Leydig cells (between tubules) with characteristic Reinke crystals
      2. May produce androgen; associated with hirsutism and virilization
   D. Fibroma
      1. Benign tumor of fibroblasts (Fig. 13.16)
      2. Associated with pleural effusions and ascites (Meigs syndrome); syndrome resolves with removal of tumor.

V. **METASTASIS**
   A. Krukenberg tumor is a metastatic mucinous tumor that involves both ovaries; most commonly due to metastatic gastric carcinoma (diffuse type)
      1. Bilaterality helps distinguish metastases from primary mucinous carcinoma of the ovary, which is usually unilateral.
   B. Pseudomyxoma peritonei is massive amounts of mucus in the peritoneum.
      1. Due to a mucinous tumor of the appendix, usually with metastasis to the ovary

GESTATIONAL PATHOLOGY

I. **ECTOPIC PREGNANCY**
   A. Implantation of fertilized ovum at a site other than the uterine wall; most common site is the lumen of the fallopian tube (Fig. 13.17).
   B. Key risk factor is scarring (e.g., secondary to pelvic inflammatory disease or endometriosis).

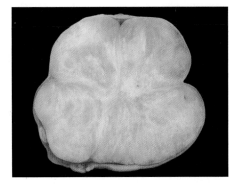

Fig. 13.16 Ovarian fibroma.

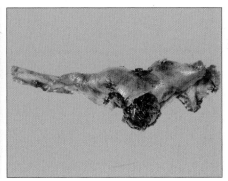

Fig. 13.17 Ectopic tubal pregnancy. (Courtesy of humpath.com)

    C. Classic presentation is lower quadrant abdominal pain a few weeks after a missed period.
        1. Surgical emergency; major complications are bleeding into fallopian tube (hematosalpinx) and rupture.

II. SPONTANEOUS ABORTION
    A. Miscarriage of fetus occurring before 20 weeks gestation (usually during first trimester)
        1. Common; occurs in up to 1/4 of recognizable pregnancies
    B. Presents as vaginal bleeding, cramp-like pain, and passage of fetal tissues
    C. Most often due to chromosomal anomalies (especially trisomy 16); other causes include hypercoagulable states (e.g., antiphospholipid syndrome), congenital infection, and exposure to teratogens (especially during the first 2 weeks of embryogenesis).
        1. Effect of teratogens generally depends on the dose, agent, and time of exposure (Table 12.1).
            i. First two weeks of gestation—spontaneous abortion
            ii. Weeks 3–8—risk of organ malformation
            iii. Months 3–9—risk of organ hypoplasia

III. PLACENTA PREVIA
    A. Implantation of the placenta in the lower uterine segment; placenta overlies cervical os (opening).
    B. Presents as third-trimester bleeding
    C. Often requires delivery of fetus by caesarian section

IV. PLACENTAL ABRUPTION
    A. Separation of placenta from the decidua prior to delivery of the fetus (Fig. 13.18)
    B. Common cause of still birth
    C. Presents with third-trimester bleeding and fetal insufficiency

V. PLACENTA ACCRETA
    A. Improper implantation of placenta into the myometrium with little or no intervening decidua
    B. Presents with difficult delivery of the placenta and postpartum bleeding

Table 12.1: Common Teratogens and Associated Effects

TERATOGEN	EFFECT
Alcohol	Most common cause of mental retardation; also leads to facial abnormalities and microcephaly
Cocaine	Intrauterine growth retardation and placental abruption
Thalidomide	Limb defects
Cigarette smoke	Intrauterine growth retardation
Isotretinoin	Spontaneous abortion, hearing and visual impairment
Tetracycline	Discolored teeth
Warfarin	Fetal bleeding
Phenytoin	Digit hypoplasia and cleft lip/palate

    C. Often requires hysterectomy

VI. PREECLAMPSIA
    A. Pregnancy-induced hypertension, proteinuria, and edema, usually arising in the third trimester; seen in approximately 5% of pregnancies
       1. Hypertension may be severe, leading to headaches and visual abnormalities.
    B. Due to abnormality of the maternal-fetal vascular interface in the placenta; resolves with delivery
    C. Eclampsia is preeclampsia with seizures.
    D. HELLP is preeclampsia with thrombotic microangiopathy involving the liver; characterized by **H**emolysis, **E**levated **L**iver enzymes, and **L**ow **P**latelets
    E. Both eclampsia and HELLP usually warrant immediate delivery.

VII. SUDDEN INFANT DEATH SYNDROME
    A. Death of a healthy infant (1 month to 1 year old) without obvious cause
    B. Infants usually expire during sleep
    C. Risk factors include sleeping on stomach, exposure to cigarette smoke, and prematurity.

VIII. HYDATIDIFORM MOLE
    A. Abnormal conception characterized by swollen and edematous villi with proliferation of trophoblasts

Table 12.2: Features of Complete and Partial Moles

	PARTIAL MOLE	COMPLETE MOLE
Genetics	Normal ovum fertilized by two sperm (or one sperm that duplicates chromosomes); 69 chromosomes	Empty ovum fertilized by two sperm (or one sperm that duplicates chromosomes); 46 chromosomes
Fetal tissue	Present	Absent
Villous edema	Some villi are hydropic, and some are normal.	Most villi are hydropic (Fig. 13.19B).
Trophoblastic proliferation	Focal proliferation present around hydropic villi	Diffuse, circumferential proliferation around hydropic villi
Risk for choriocarcinoma	Minimal	2–3%

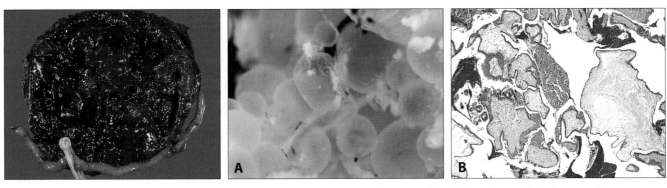

Fig. 13.18 Placental abruption. (Courtesy of Jerome Taxy, MD)

Fig. 13.19 Complete mole. **A**, Swollen, 'grape-like' villi. **B**, Hydropic villi. (A, Courtesy of Steven O'Connor, MD)

B. Uterus expands as if a normal pregnancy is present, but the uterus is much larger and β-hCG much higher than expected for date of gestation.

C. Classically presents in the second trimester as passage of grape-like masses through the vaginal canal (Fig. 13.19A).

1. With prenatal care, moles are diagnosed by routine ultrasound in the early first trimester. Fetal heart sounds are absent, and a 'snowstorm' appearance is classically seen on ultrasound.

D. Classified as complete or partial (Table 12.2)

E. Treatment is suction curettage.

1. Subsequent β-hCG monitoring is important to ensure adequate mole removal and to screen for the development of choriocarcinoma.

   i. Choriocarcinoma may arise as a complication of gestation (spontaneous abortion, normal pregnancy, or hydatidiform mole) or as a spontaneous germ cell tumor.

   ii. Choriocarcinomas that arise from the gestational pathway respond well to chemotherapy; those that arise from the germ cell pathway do not.

REMINDER

Thank you for choosing Pathoma for your studies. We strive to provide the highest quality educational materials while keeping affordability in mind. A tremendous amount of time and effort has gone into developing these materials, so we appreciate your legitimate use of this program. It speaks to your integrity as a future physician and the high ethical standards that we all set forth for ourselves when taking the Hippocratic oath. Unauthorized use of Pathoma materials is contrary to the ethical standards of a training physician and is a violation of copyright. Pathoma videos are updated on a regular basis and the most current version, as well as a complete list of errata, can be accessed through your account at Pathoma.com.

Sincerely,

Dr. Sattar, MD

Male Genital System Pathology

14

PENIS

I. **HYPOSPADIAS**
   A. Opening of urethra on inferior surface of penis
   B. Due to failure of the urethral folds to close

II. **EPISPADIAS**
   A. Opening of urethra on superior surface of penis
   B. Due to abnormal positioning of the genital tubercle
   C. Associated with bladder exstrophy

III. **CONDYLOMA ACUMINATUM**
   A. Benign warty growth on genital skin
   B. Due to HPV type 6 or 11; characterized by koilocytic change (Fig. 14.1)

IV. **LYMPHOGRANULOMA VENEREUM**
   A. Necrotizing granulomatous inflammation of the inguinal lymphatics and lymph nodes
   B. Sexually transmitted disease caused by *Chlamydia trachomatis* (serotypes L1-L3)
   C. Eventually heals with fibrosis; perianal involvement may result in rectal stricture.

V. **SQUAMOUS CELL CARCINOMA**
   A. Malignant proliferation of squamous cells of penile skin
   B. Risk factors
      1. High risk HPV (2/3 of cases)
      2. Lack of circumcision—Foreskin acts as a nidus for inflammation and irritation if not properly maintained.
   C. Precursor in situ lesions
      1. Bowen disease—in situ carcinoma of the penile shaft or scrotum that presents as leukoplakia
      2. Erythroplasia of Queyrat—in situ carcinoma on the glans that presents as erythroplakia
      3. Bowenoid papulosis—in situ carcinoma that presents as multiple reddish papules
         i. Seen in younger patients (40s) relative to Bowen disease and erythroplasia of Queyrat
         ii. Does not progress to invasive carcinoma

TESTICLE

I. **CRYPTORCHIDISM**
   A. Failure of testicle to descend into the scrotal sac
      1. Testicles normally develop in the abdomen and then "descend" into the scrotal sac as the fetus grows.
   B. Most common congenital male reproductive abnormality; seen in 1% of male infants

C. Most cases resolve spontaneously; otherwise, orchiopexy is performed before 2 years of age.

D. Complications include testicular atrophy with infertility and increased risk for seminoma.

II. ORCHITIS

A. Inflammation of the testicle

B. Causes

1. *Chlamydia trachomatis* (serotypes D-K) or *Neisseria gonorrhoeae*—Seen in young adults. Increased risk of sterility, but libido is not affected because Leydig cells are spared.

2. *Escherichia coli* and *Pseudomonas*—Seen in older adults; urinary tract infection pathogens spread into the reproductive tract.

3. Mumps virus (teenage males)—increased risk for infertility; testicular inflammation is usually not seen in children < 10 years old.

4. Autoimmune orchitis—characterized by granulomas involving the seminiferous tubules

III. TESTICULAR TORSION

A. Twisting of the spermatic cord; thin-walled veins become obstructed leading to congestion and hemorrhagic infarction (Fig. 14.2).

B. Usually due to congenital failure of testes to attach to the inner lining of the scrotum (via the processus vaginalis)

C. Presents in adolescents with sudden testicular pain and absent cremasteric reflex

IV. VARICOCELE

A. Dilation of the spermatic vein due to impaired drainage

B. Presents as scrotal swelling with a "bag of worms" appearance

C. Usually left sided; left testicular vein drains into the left renal vein, while the right testicular vein drains directly into the IVC.

1. Associated with left-sided renal cell carcinoma; RCC often invades the renal vein.

D. Seen in a large percentage of infertile males

V. HYDROCELE

A. Fluid collection within the tunica vaginalis

1. Tunica vaginalis is a serous membrane that covers the testicle as well as the internal surface of the scrotum.

B. Associated with incomplete closure of the processus vaginalis leading to communication with the peritoneal cavity (infants) or blockage of lymphatic drainage (adults)

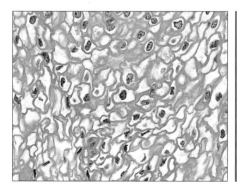

Fig. 14.1 Koilocytic change.

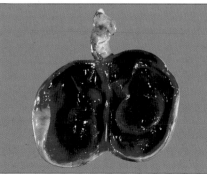

Fig. 14.2 Hemorrhagic infarction of testicle. (Courtesy of humpath.com)

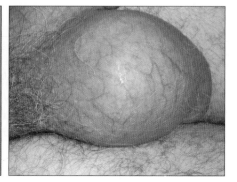

Fig. 14.3 Hydrocele.

C. Presents as scrotal swelling that can be transilluminated (Fig. 14.3)

TESTICULAR TUMORS

I. **BASIC PRINCIPLES**
   A. Arise from germ cells or sex cord-stroma
   B. Present as a firm, painless testicular mass that cannot be transilluminated
   C. Usually not biopsied due to risk of seeding the scrotum; removed via radical orchiectomy
      1. Most testicular tumors are malignant germ cell tumors.

II. **GERM CELL TUMORS**
   A. Most common type of testicular tumor (> 95% of cases)
   B. Usually occur between 15–40 years of age
   C. Risk factors include cryptorchidism and Klinefelter syndrome.
   D. Divided into seminoma and nonseminoma
      1. Seminomas (55% of cases) are highly responsive to radiotherapy, metastasize late, and have an excellent prognosis.
      2. Nonseminomas (45% of cases) show variable response to treatment and often metastasize early.
   E. Seminoma is a malignant tumor comprised of large cells with clear cytoplasm and central nuclei (resemble spermatogonia, Fig. 14.4A); forms a homogeneous mass with no hemorrhage or necrosis (Fig. 14.4B)
      1. Most common testicular tumor; resembles ovarian dysgerminoma
      2. Rare cases may produce β-hCG.
      3. Good prognosis; responds to radiotherapy
   F. Embryonal carcinoma is a malignant tumor comprised of immature, primitive cells that may produce glands (Fig. 14.5A); forms a hemorrhagic mass with necrosis (Fig. 14.5B)
      1. Aggressive with early hematogenous spread
      2. Chemotherapy may result in differentiation into another type of germ cell tumor (e.g., teratoma).
      3. Increased AFP or β-hCG may be present.
   G. Yolk sac (endodermal sinus) tumor is a malignant tumor that resembles yolk sac elements.
      1. Most common testicular tumor in children
      2. Schiller-Duval bodies (glomerulus-like structures) are seen on histology (Fig. 14.6).
      3. AFP is characteristically elevated.

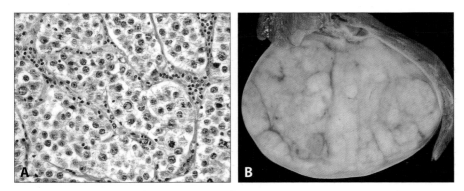

Fig. 14.4 Seminoma. **A,** Microscopic appearance. **B,** Gross appearance. (A, Courtesy of Ed Uthman, MD)

H. Choriocarcinoma is a malignant tumor of syncytiotrophoblasts and cytotrophoblasts (placenta-like tissue, but villi are absent, Fig. 14.7).
   1. Spreads early via blood
   2. β-hCG is characteristically elevated; may lead to hyperthyroidism or gynecomastia (α-subunit of hCG is similar to that of FSH, LH, and TSH)
I. Teratoma is a tumor composed of mature fetal tissue derived from two or three embryonic layers.
   1. Malignant in males (as opposed to females)
   2. AFP or β-hCG may be increased.
J. Mixed germ cell tumors
   1. Germ cell tumors are usually mixed.
   2. Prognosis is based on the worst component.

III. SEX CORD–STROMAL TUMORS

A. Tumors that resemble sex cord-stromal tissues of the testicle (Fig. 14.8); usually benign
B. Leydig cell tumor usually produces androgen, causing precocious puberty in children or gynecomastia in adults.
   1. Characteristic Reinke crystals may be seen on histology.
C. Sertoli cell tumor is comprised of tubules and is usually clinically silent.

IV. LYMPHOMA

A. Most common cause of a testicular mass in males > 60 years old; often bilateral
B. Usually of diffuse large B-cell type

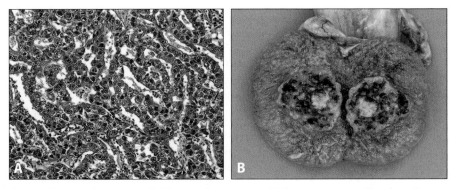

Fig. 14.5 Embryonal carcinoma. **A**, Microscopic appearance. **B**, Gross appearance. (Courtesy of webpathology.com)

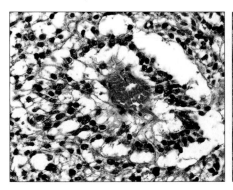

Fig. 14.6 Schiller-Duval body, yolk sac tumor. (Courtesy of webpathology.com)

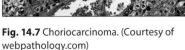

Fig. 14.7 Choriocarcinoma. (Courtesy of webpathology.com)

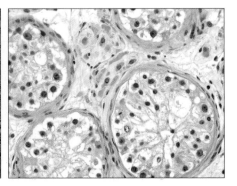

Fig. 14.8 Normal testicle, microscopic appearance.

PROSTATE

I. **BASIC PRINCIPLES**
   A. Small, round organ that lies at the base of the bladder encircling the urethra
   B. Sits anterior to the rectum; posterior aspect of prostate is palpable by digital rectal exam (DRE).
   C. Consists of glands and stroma (Fig. 14.9)
      1. Glands are composed of an inner layer of luminal cells and an outer layer of basal cells; secrete alkaline, milky fluid that is added to sperm and seminal vesicle fluid to make semen.
      2. Glands and stroma are maintained by androgens.

II. **ACUTE PROSTATITIS**
   A. Acute inflammation of the prostate; usually due to bacteria
      1. *Chlamydia trachomatis* and *Neisseria gonorrhoeae* are common causes in young adults.
      2. *Escherichia coli* and *Pseudomonas* are common causes in older adults.
   B. Presents as dysuria with fever and chills
   C. Prostate is tender and boggy on digital rectal exam.
   D. Prostatic secretions show WBCs; culture reveals bacteria.

III. **CHRONIC PROSTATITIS**
   A. Chronic inflammation of prostate
   B. Presents as dysuria with pelvic or low back pain
   C. Prostatic secretions show WBCs, but cultures are negative.

IV. **BENIGN PROSTATIC HYPERPLASIA (BPH)**
   A. Hyperplasia of prostatic stroma and glands
   B. Age-related change (present in most men by the age of 60 years); no increased risk for cancer
   C. Related to dihydrotestosterone (DHT)
      1. Testosterone is converted to DHT by 5α-reductase in stromal cells.
      2. DHT acts on the androgen receptor of stromal and epithelial cells resulting in hyperplastic nodules.
   D. Occurs in the central periurethral zone of the prostate
   E. Clinical features include
      1. Problems starting and stopping urine stream
      2. Impaired bladder emptying with increased risk for infection and hydronephrosis (Fig. 14.10)
      3. Dribbling

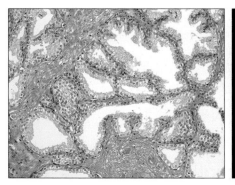

Fig. 14.9 Normal prostate, microscopic appearance.

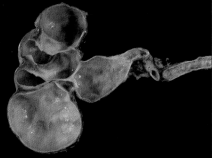

Fig. 14.10 Hydronephrosis.

4. Hypertrophy of bladder wall smooth muscle; increased risk for bladder diverticula

5. Microscopic hematuria may be present.

6. Prostate-specific antigen (PSA) is often slightly elevated (usually less than 10 ng/mL) due to the increased number of glands; PSA is made by prostatic glands and liquefies semen.

F. Treatment

1. α_1-antagonist (e.g., terazosin) to relax smooth muscle

    i. Also relaxes vascular smooth muscle lowering blood pressure

    ii. Selective α_{1A}-antagonists (e.g., tamsulosin) are used in normotensive individuals to avoid α_{1B} effects on blood vessels.

2. 5α-reductase inhibitor

    i. Blocks conversion of testosterone to DHT

    ii. Takes months to produce results

    iii. Also useful for male pattern baldness

    iv. Side effects are gynecomastia and sexual dysfunction.

V. **PROSTATE ADENOCARCINOMA**

A. Malignant proliferation of prostatic glands

B. Most common cancer in men; 2nd most common cause of cancer-related death

C. Risk factors include age, race (African Americans > Caucasians > Asians), and diet high in saturated fats.

D. Prostatic carcinoma is most often clinically silent.

1. Usually arises in the peripheral, posterior region of the prostate and, hence, does not produce urinary symptoms early on (Fig. 14.11A)

2. Screening begins at the age of 50 years with DRE and PSA.

    i. Normal serum PSA increases with age due to BPH (2.5 ng/mL for ages 40–49 years vs. 7.5 ng/mL for ages 70 – 79 years)

    ii. PSA > 10 ng/mL is highly worrisome at any age.

    iii. Decreased % free-PSA is suggestive of cancer (cancer makes bound PSA).

E. Prostatic biopsy is required to confirm the presence of carcinoma.

1. Shows small, invasive glands with prominent nucleoli (Fig. 14.11B)

2. Gleason grading system is based on architecture alone (and not nuclear atypia).

    i. Multiple regions of the tumor are assessed because architecture varies from area to area.

    ii. A score (1–5) is assigned for two distinct areas and then added to produce a final score (2–10).

    iii. Higher score suggests worse prognosis.

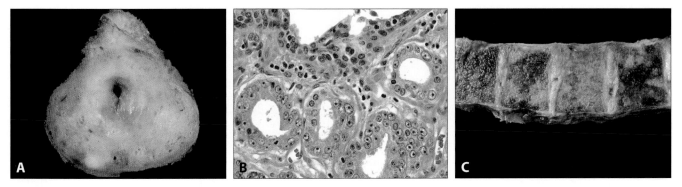

Fig. 14.11 Prostatic adenocarcinoma. **A,** Gross appearance. **B,** Microscopic appearance. **C,** Osteoblastic metastasis involving lumbar spine.

F. Spread to lumbar spine or pelvis is common (Fig. 14.11C); results in osteoblastic metastases that present as low back pain and increased serum alkaline phosphatase, PSA, and prostatic acid phosphatase (PAP)

G. Prostatectomy is performed for localized disease; advanced disease is treated with hormone suppression to reduce testosterone and DHT.

   1. Continuous GnRH analogs (e.g., leuprolide) shut down the anterior pituitary gonadotrophs (LH and FSH are reduced).

   2. Flutamide acts as a competitive inhibitor at the androgen receptor.

Endocrine Pathology

15

INTRODUCTION

I. **ENDOCRINE SYSTEM**
   A. Group of glands that maintain body homeostasis
   B. Functions by release of hormones that travel via blood to distant organs
   C. "Feedback" mechanisms control hormone release.

ANTERIOR PITUITARY GLAND

I. **PITUITARY ADENOMA**
   A. Benign tumor of anterior pituitary cells
   B. May be functional (hormone-producing) or nonfunctional (silent)
      1. Nonfunctional tumors often present with mass effect.
         i. Bitemporal hemianopsia occurs due to compression of the optic chiasm.
         ii. Hypopituitarism occurs due to compression of normal pituitary tissue.
         iii. Headache
      2. Functional tumors present with features based on the type of hormone produced.
   C. Prolactinoma presents as galactorrhea and amenorrhea (females) or as decreased libido and headache (males); most common type of pituitary adenoma
      1. Treatment is dopamine agonists (e.g., bromocriptine or cabergoline) to suppress prolactin production (shrinks tumor) or surgery for larger lesions.
   D. Growth hormone cell adenoma
      1. Gigantism in children—increased linear bone growth (epiphyses are not fused)
      2. Acromegaly in adults
         i. Enlarged bones of hands, feet, and jaw
         ii. Growth of visceral organs leading to dysfunction (e.g., cardiac failure)
         iii. Enlarged tongue
      3. Secondary diabetes mellitus is often present (GH induces liver gluconeogenesis).
      4. Diagnosed by elevated GH and insulin growth factor-1 (IGF-1) levels along with lack of GH suppression by oral glucose
      5. Treatment is octreotide (somatostatin analog that suppresses GH release), GH receptor antagonists, or surgery.
   E. ACTH cell adenomas secrete ACTH leading to Cushing syndrome (see "Adrenal Cortex" below).
   F. TSH cell, LH-producing, and FSH-producing adenomas occur, but are rare.

II. **HYPOPITUITARISM**
   A. Insufficient production of hormones by the anterior pituitary gland; symptoms arise when > 75% of the pituitary parenchyma is lost.
   B. Causes include
      1. Pituitary adenomas (adults) or craniopharyngioma (children)—due to mass effect or pituitary apoplexy (bleeding into an adenoma)
      2. Sheehan syndrome—pregnancy-related infarction of the pituitary gland
         i. Gland doubles in size during pregnancy, but blood supply does not increase significantly; blood loss during parturition precipitates infarction.

      ii. Presents as poor lactation, loss of pubic hair, and fatigue
   3. Empty sella syndrome—congenital defect of the sella
      i. Herniation of the arachnoid and CSF into the sella compresses and destroys the pituitary gland.
      ii. Pituitary gland is "absent" (empty sella) on imaging.

POSTERIOR PITUITARY GLAND

I. **BASIC PRINCIPLES**
  A. Antidiuretic hormone (ADH) and oxytocin are made in the hypothalamus and then transported via axons to the posterior pituitary for release.
    1. ADH acts on the distal tubules and collecting ducts of the kidney to promote free water retention.
    2. Oxytocin mediates uterine contraction during labor and release of breast milk (let-down) in lactating mothers.

II. **CENTRAL DIABETES INSIPIDUS**
  A. ADH deficiency
  B. Due to hypothalamic or posterior pituitary pathology (e.g., tumor, trauma, infection, or inflammation)
  C. Clinical features are based on loss of free water.
    1. Polyuria and polydipsia with risk of life-threatening dehydration
    2. Hypernatremia and high serum osmolality
    3. Low urine osmolality and specific gravity
  D. Water deprivation test fails to increase urine osmolality (useful for diagnosis).
  E. Treatment is desmopressin (ADH analog).

III. **NEPHROGENIC DIABETES INSIPIDUS**
  A. Impaired renal response to ADH
  B. Due to inherited mutations or drugs (e.g., lithium and demeclocycline)
  C. Clinical features are similar to central diabetes insipidus, but there is no response to desmopressin.

IV. **SYNDROME OF INAPPROPRIATE ADH (SIADH) SECRETION**
  A. Excessive ADH secretion
  B. Most often due to ectopic production (e.g., small cell carcinoma of the lung); other causes include CNS trauma, pulmonary infection, and drugs (e.g., cyclophosphamide).
  C. Clinical features are based on retention of free water.
    1. Hyponatremia and low serum osmolality
    2. Mental status changes and seizures—Hyponatremia leads to neuronal swelling and cerebral edema.
  D. Treatment is free water restriction or demeclocycline.

THYROID GLAND

I. **THYROGLOSSAL DUCT CYST**
  A. Cystic dilation of thyroglossal duct remnant
    1. Thyroid develops at the base of tongue and then travels along the thyroglossal duct to the anterior neck.
    2. Thyroglossal duct normally involutes; a persistent duct, however, may undergo cystic dilation.
  B. Presents as an anterior neck mass

II. **LINGUAL THYROID**

A. Persistence of thyroid tissue at the base of tongue

B. Presents as a base of tongue mass

HYPERTHYROIDISM

I. **BASIC PRINCIPLES**

A. Increased level of circulating thyroid hormone

1. Increases basal metabolic rate (due to increased synthesis of Na^+-K^+ ATPase)

2. Increases sympathetic nervous system activity (due to increased expression of β_1-adrenergic receptors)

B. Clinical features include

1. Weight loss despite increased appetite

2. Heat intolerance and sweating

3. Tachycardia with increased cardiac output

4. Arrhythmia (e.g., atrial fibrillation), especially in the elderly

5. Tremor, anxiety, insomnia, and heightened emotions

6. Staring gaze with lid lag

7. Diarrhea with malabsorption

8. Oligomenorrhea

9. Bone resorption with hypercalcemia (risk for osteoporosis)

10. Decreased muscle mass with weakness

11. Hypocholesterolemia

12. Hyperglycemia (due to gluconeogenesis and glycogenolysis)

II. **GRAVES DISEASE**

A. Autoantibody (IgG) that stimulates TSH receptor (type II hypersensitivity)

B. Leads to increased synthesis and release of thyroid hormone

1. Most common cause of hyperthyroidism

2. Classically occurs in women of childbearing age (20–40 years)

C. Clinical features include

1. Hyperthyroidism

2. Diffuse goiter—Constant TSH stimulation leads to thyroid hyperplasia and hypertrophy (Fig. 15.1A).

3. Exophthalmos and pretibial myxedema

i. Fibroblasts behind the orbit and overlying the shin express the TSH receptor.

ii. TSH activation results in glycosaminoglycan (chondroitin sulfate and hyaluronic acid) buildup, inflammation, fibrosis, and edema leading to exophthalmos and pretibial myxedema.

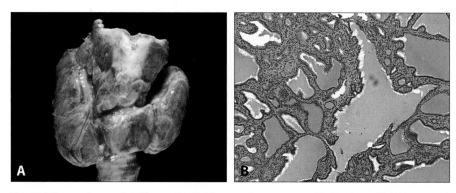

Fig. 15.1 Graves disease. **A**, Diffuse goiter. **B**, Microscopic appearance. (A, Courtesy of Ed Uthman, MD)

    D. Irregular follicles with scalloped colloid and chronic inflammation are seen on histology (Fig. 15.1B).

    E. Laboratory findings include

       1. ↑ total and free T_4; ↓ TSH (free T_3 downregulates TRH receptors in the anterior pituitary to decrease TSH release)

       2. Hypocholesterolemia

       3. Increased serum glucose

    F. Treatment involves β-blockers, thioamide, and radioiodine ablation.

    G. Thyroid storm is a potentially fatal complication.

       1. Due to elevated catecholamines and massive hormone excess, usually in response to stress (e.g., surgery or childbirth)

       2. Presents as arrhythmia, hyperthermia, and vomiting with hypovolemic shock

       3. Treatment is propylthiouracil (PTU), β-blockers, and steroids.

          i. PTU inhibits peroxidase-mediated oxidation, organification, and coupling steps of thyroid hormone synthesis, as well as peripheral conversion of T_4 to T_3.

III. MULTINODULAR GOITER

    A. Enlarged thyroid gland with multiple nodules (Fig. 15.2)

    B. Due to relative iodine deficiency

    C. Usually nontoxic (euthyroid)

    D. Rarely, regions become TSH-independent leading to T_4 release and hyperthyroidism ('toxic goiter').

HYPOTHYROIDISM

I. CRETINISM

    A. Hypothyroidism in neonates and infants

    B. Characterized by mental retardation, short stature with skeletal abnormalities, coarse facial features, enlarged tongue, and umbilical hernia

       1. Thyroid hormone is required for normal brain and skeletal development.

    C. Causes include maternal hypothyroidism during early pregnancy, thyroid agenesis, dyshormonogenetic goiter, and iodine deficiency.

       1. Dyshormonogenetic goiter is due to a congenital defect in thyroid hormone production; most commonly involves thyroid peroxidase

II. MYXEDEMA

    A. Hypothyroidism in older children or adults

    B. Clinical features are based on decreased basal metabolic rate and decreased sympathetic nervous system activity.

       1. Myxedema—accumulation of glycosaminoglycans in the skin and soft tissue; results in a deepening of voice and large tongue

       2. Weight gain despite normal appetite

       3. Slowing of mental activity

       4. Muscle weakness

       5. Cold intolerance with decreased sweating

       6. Bradycardia with decreased cardiac output, leading to shortness of breath and fatigue

       7. Oligomenorrhea

       8. Hypercholesterolemia

       9. Constipation

    C. Most common causes are iodine deficiency and Hashimoto thyroiditis; other causes include drugs (e.g., lithium) and surgical removal or radioablation of the thyroid.

THYROIDITIS

I. **HASHIMOTO THYROIDITIS**
   A. Autoimmune destruction of the thyroid gland; associated with HLA-DR5
      1. Most common cause of hypothyroidism in regions where iodine levels are adequate
   B. Clinical features
      1. Initially may present as hyperthyroidism (due to follicle damage)
      2. Progresses to hypothyroidism; $\downarrow T_4$ and $\uparrow$ TSH
      3. Antithyroglobulin and antithyroid peroxidase antibodies are often present (sign of thyroid damage).
   C. Chronic inflammation with germinal centers and Hurthle cells (eosinophilic metaplasia of cells that line follicles) is seen on histology (Fig. 15.3).
   D. Increased risk for B-cell (marginal zone) lymphoma; presents as an enlarging thyroid gland late in disease course

II. **SUBACUTE GRANULOMATOUS (DE QUERVAIN) THYROIDITIS**
   A. Granulomatous thyroiditis that follows a viral infection
   B. Presents as a tender thyroid with transient hyperthyroidism
   C. Self-limited; rarely (15% of cases) may progress to hypothyroidism

III. **REIDEL FIBROSING THYROIDITIS**
   A. Chronic inflammation with extensive fibrosis of the thyroid gland
   B. Presents as hypothyroidism with a 'hard as wood,' nontender thyroid gland
   C. Fibrosis may extend to involve local structures (e.g., airway).
      1. Clinically mimics anaplastic carcinoma, but patients are younger (40s), and malignant cells are absent

THYROID NEOPLASIA

I. **BASIC PRINCIPLES**
   A. Usually presents as a distinct, solitary nodule
      1. Thyroid nodules are more likely to be benign than malignant.
   B. ^{131}I radioactive uptake studies are useful to further characterize nodules.
      1. Increased uptake ('hot' nodule) is seen in Graves disease or nodular goiter.
      2. Decreased uptake ('cold' nodule) is seen in adenoma and carcinoma; often warrants biopsy
   C. Biopsy is performed by fine needle aspiration (FNA).

II. **FOLLICULAR ADENOMA**
   A. Benign proliferation of follicles surrounded by a fibrous capsule (Fig. 15.4)

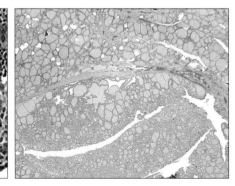

Fig. 15.2 Multinodular goiter. (Courtesy of Jamie Steinmetz, MD)   **Fig. 15.3** Hashimoto thyroiditis.   **Fig. 15.4** Follicular adenoma.

B. Usually nonfunctional; less commonly, may secrete thyroid hormone

III. **PAPILLARY CARCINOMA**
   A. Most common type of thyroid carcinoma (80% of cases)
   B. Exposure to ionizing radiation in childhood is a major risk factor.
   C. Comprised of papillae lined by cells with clear, 'Orphan Annie eye' nuclei and nuclear grooves (Fig. 15.5A); papillae are often associated with psammoma bodies (Fig. 15.5B).
   D. Often spreads to cervical (neck) lymph nodes, but prognosis is excellent (10-year survival > 95%)

IV. **FOLLICULAR CARCINOMA**
   A. Malignant proliferation of follicles surrounded by a fibrous capsule with invasion through the capsule (Fig. 15.6)
      1. Invasion through the capsule helps distinguish follicular carcinoma from follicular adenoma.
      2. Entire capsule must be examined microscopically.
      3. FNA only examines cells and not the capsule; hence, a distinction between follicular adenoma and follicular carcinoma cannot be made by FNA.
   B. Metastasis generally occurs hematogenously.

V. **MEDULLARY CARCINOMA**
   A. Malignant proliferation of parafollicular C cells; comprises 5% of thyroid carcinomas
      1. C cells are neuroendocrine cells that secrete calcitonin.
      2. Calcitonin lowers serum calcium by increasing renal calcium excretion but is inactive at normal physiologic levels.
      3. High levels of calcitonin produced by tumor may lead to hypocalcemia.
      4. Calcitonin often deposits within the tumor as amyloid.
   B. Biopsy reveals sheets of malignant cells in an amyloid stroma (Fig. 15.7).
   C. Familial cases are often due to multiple endocrine neoplasia (MEN) 2A and 2B, which are associated with mutations in the *RET* oncogene.
      1. MEN 2 results in medullary carcinoma, pheochromocytoma, and parathyroid adenomas (2A) or ganglioneuromas of the oral mucosa (2B).
      2. Detection of the *RET* mutation warrants prophylactic thyroidectomy.

VI. **ANAPLASTIC CARCINOMA**
   A. Undifferentiated malignant tumor of the thyroid (Fig. 15.8); usually seen in elderly
   B. Often invades local structures, leading to dysphagia or respiratory compromise
   C. Poor prognosis

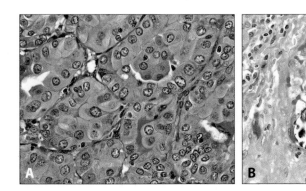

Fig. 15.5 Papillary carcinoma. **A**, Nuclear features. **B**, Psammoma bodies.

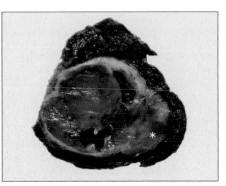

Fig. 15.6 Follicular carcinoma. (Courtesy of Bulent Celasun, MD)

PARATHYROID GLANDS

I. **BASIC PRINCIPLES**

    A. Chief cells regulate serum free (ionized) calcium via parathyroid hormone (PTH) secretion, which

        1. Increases bone osteoclast activity, releasing calcium and phosphate

        2. Increases small bowel absorption of calcium and phosphate (indirectly by activating vitamin D)

        3. Increases renal calcium reabsorption (distal tubule) and decreases phosphate reabsorption (proximal tubule)

    B. Increased serum ionized calcium levels provide negative feedback to decrease PTH secretion.

II. **PRIMARY HYPERPARATHYROIDISM**

    A. Excess PTH due to a disorder of the parathyroid gland itself

    B. Most common cause is parathyroid adenoma (>80% of cases); sporadic parathyroid hyperplasia and parathyroid carcinoma are less common causes.

    C. Parathyroid adenoma is a benign neoplasm, usually involving one gland.

        1. Most often results in asymptomatic hypercalcemia; however, may present with consequences of increased PTH and hypercalcemia such as

            i. Nephrolithiasis (calcium oxalate stones)

            ii. Nephrocalcinosis—metastatic calcification of renal tubules (Fig. 15.9), potentially leading to renal insufficiency and polyuria

            iii. CNS disturbances (e.g., depression and seizures)

            iv. Constipation, peptic ulcer disease, and acute pancreatitis

            v. Osteitis fibrosa cystica—resorption of bone leading to fibrosis and cystic spaces (Fig. 15.10)

        2. Laboratory findings include ↑ serum PTH, ↑ serum calcium, ↓ serum phosphate, ↑ urinary cAMP, and ↑ serum alkaline phosphatase.

        3. Treatment involves surgical removal of the affected gland.

III. **SECONDARY HYPERPARATHYROIDISM**

    A. Excess production of PTH due to a disease process extrinsic to the parathyroid gland

    B. Most common cause is chronic renal failure.

        1. Renal insufficiency leads to decreased phosphate excretion.

        2. ↑ serum phosphate binds free calcium.

        3. ↓ free calcium stimulates all four parathyroid glands.

        4. ↑ PTH leads to bone resorption (contributing to renal osteodystrophy).

        5. Lab findings include ↑ PTH, ↓ serum calcium, ↑ serum phosphate, and ↑ alkaline phosphatase.

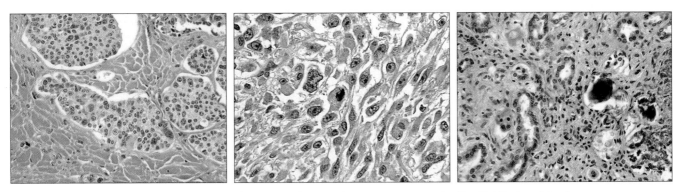

Fig. 15.7 Medullary carcinoma.   **Fig. 15.8** Anaplastic carcinoma.   **Fig. 15.9** Nephrocalcinosis.

IV. **HYPOPARATHYROIDISM**

    A. Low PTH

    B. Causes include autoimmune damage to the parathyroids, surgical excision, and DiGeorge syndrome

    C. Presents with symptoms related to low serum calcium

        1. Numbness and tingling (particularly circumoral)

        2. Muscle spasms (tetany)—may be elicited with filling of a blood pressure cuff (Trousseau sign) or tapping on the facial nerve (Chvostek sign)

    D. Labs reveal ↓ PTH levels and ↓ serum calcium.

    E. Pseudohypoparathyroidism is due to end-organ resistance to PTH.

        1. Labs reveal hypocalcemia with ↑ PTH levels.

        2. Autosomal dominant form is associated with short stature and short 4th and 5th digits.

ENDOCRINE PANCREAS

I. **BASIC PRINCIPLES**

    A. Composed of clusters of cells termed islets of Langerhans (Fig. 15.11)

    B. A single islet consists of multiple cell types, each producing one type of hormone.

    C. Insulin is secreted by beta cells, which lie in the center of the islets.

        1. Major anabolic hormone; upregulates insulin-dependent glucose transporter protein (GLUT4) on skeletal muscle and adipose tissue (glucose uptake by GLUT4 decreases serum glucose)

        2. Increased glucose uptake by tissues leads to increased glycogen synthesis, protein synthesis, and lipogenesis.

    D. Glucagon is secreted by alpha cells; it opposes insulin in order to increase blood glucose levels (e.g., in states of fasting) via glycogenolysis and lipolysis.

II. **TYPE 1 DIABETES MELLITUS**

    A. Insulin deficiency leading to a metabolic disorder characterized by hyperglycemia

    B. Due to autoimmune destruction of beta cells by T lymphocytes

        1. Characterized by inflammation of islets

        2. Associated with HLA-DR3 and HLA-DR4

        3. Autoantibodies against insulin are often present (sign of damage) and may be seen years before clinical disease develops.

    C. Manifests in childhood with clinical features of insulin deficiency

        1. High serum glucose—Lack of insulin leads to decreased glucose uptake by fat and skeletal muscle.

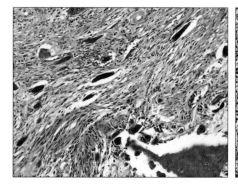

Fig. 15.10 Osteitis fibrosa cystica.

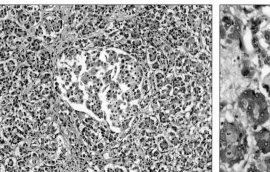

Fig. 15.11 Islets of Langerhans.

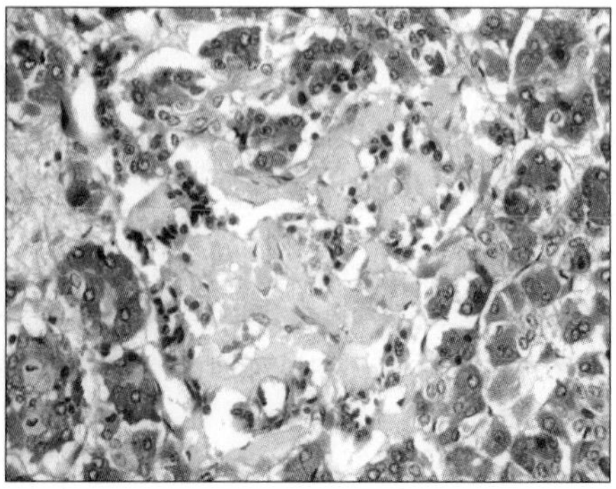

Fig. 15.12 Amyloid in islets, type II DM.

2. Weight loss, low muscle mass, and polyphagia—Unopposed glucagon leads to gluconeogenesis, glycogenolysis and lipolysis, which further exacerbates hyperglycemia.

3. Polyuria, polydipsia, and glycosuria—Hyperglycemia exceeds renal ability to resorb glucose; excess filtered glucose leads to osmotic diuresis.

4. Treatment involves lifelong insulin.

D. Risk for diabetic ketoacidosis

1. Characterized by excessive serum ketones

2. Often arises with stress (e.g., infection); epinephrine stimulates glucagon secretion increasing lipolysis (along with gluconeogenesis and glycogenolysis).
   i. Increased lipolysis leads to increased free fatty acids (FFAs).
   ii. Liver converts FFAs to ketone bodies (β-hydroxybutyric acid and acetoacetic acid).

3. Results in hyperglycemia (> 300 mg/dL), anion gap metabolic acidosis, and hyperkalemia

4. Presents with Kussmaul respirations, dehydration, nausea, vomiting, mental status changes, and fruity smelling breath (due to acetone)

5. Treatment is fluids (corrects dehydration from polyuria), insulin, and replacement of electrolytes (e.g., potassium).

III. TYPE 2 DIABETES MELLITUS

A. End-organ insulin resistance leading to a metabolic disorder characterized by hyperglycemia

1. Most common type of diabetes (90% of cases); affects 5–10% of the US population

2. Incidence is rising.

B. Arises in middle-aged, obese adults

1. Obesity leads to decreased numbers of insulin receptors.

2. Strong genetic predisposition exists.

C. Insulin levels are increased early in disease, but later, insulin deficiency develops due to beta cell exhaustion; histology reveals amyloid deposition in the islets (Fig. 15.12).

D. Clinical features include polyuria, polydipsia, and hyperglycemia, but disease is often clinically silent.

E. Diagnosis is made by measuring glucose levels (normal is 70–120 mg/dL).

1. Random glucose > 200 mg/dL

2. Fasting glucose > 126 mg/dL

3. Glucose tolerance test with a serum glucose level > 200 mg/dL two hours after glucose loading

F. Treatment involves weight loss (diet and exercise) initially; may require drug therapy to counter insulin resistance (e.g., sulfonylureas or metformin) or exogenous insulin after exhaustion of beta cells

G. Risk for hyperosmolar non-ketotic coma

1. High glucose (> 500 mg/dL) leads to life-threatening diuresis with hypotension and coma.

2. Ketones are absent due to small amounts of circulating insulin.

IV. LONG-TERM CONSEQUENCES OF DIABETES

A. Nonenzymatic glycosylation (NEG) of vascular basement membranes

1. NEG of large- and medium-sized vessels leads to atherosclerosis and its resultant complications.
   i. Cardiovascular disease is the leading cause of death among diabetics.
   ii. Peripheral vascular disease in diabetics is the leading cause of nontraumatic amputations.

2. NEG of small vessels (arterioles) leads to hyaline arteriolosclerosis (Fig. 15.13A).
    i. Involvement of renal arterioles leads to glomerulosclerosis, resulting in small, scarred kidneys with a granular surface (Fig. 15.13B).
    ii. Preferential involvement of efferent arterioles leads to glomerular hyperfiltration injury with microalbuminuria that eventually progresses to nephrotic syndrome; characterized by Kimmelstiel-Wilson nodules in glomeruli
3. NEG of hemoglobin produces glycated hemoglobin (HbA_{1C}), a marker of glycemic control.

B. Osmotic damage
1. Glucose freely enters into Schwann cells (which myelinate peripheral nerves), pericytes of retinal blood vessels, and the lens.
2. Aldose reductase converts glucose to sorbitol, resulting in osmotic damage.
3. Leads to peripheral neuropathy, impotence, blindness, and cataracts; diabetes is the leading cause of blindness in the developed world.

V. PANCREATIC ENDOCRINE NEOPLASMS

A. Tumors of islet cells; account for < 5% of pancreatic neoplasms.
1. Often a component of MEN 1 along with parathyroid hyperplasia and pituitary adenomas
B. Insulinomas present as episodic hypoglycemia with mental status changes that are relieved by administration of glucose.
1. Diagnosed by ↓ serum glucose levels (usually < 50 mg/dL), ↑ insulin, and ↑ C-peptide
C. Gastrinomas present as treatment-resistant peptic ulcers (Zollinger-Ellison syndrome); ulcers may be multiple and can extend into the jejunum.
D. Somatostatinomas present as achlorhydria (due to inhibition of gastrin) and cholelithiasis with steatorrhea (due to inhibition of cholecystokinin).
E. VIPomas secrete excessive vasoactive intestinal peptide leading to watery diarrhea, hypokalemia, and achlorhydria.

ADRENAL CORTEX

I. BASIC PRINCIPLES

A. Composed of three layers that each secrete distinct hormones
1. Glomerulosa produces mineralocorticoids (e.g., aldosterone).
2. Fasciculata produces glucocorticoids (e.g., cortisol).
3. Reticularis produces sex steroids (e.g., testosterone).

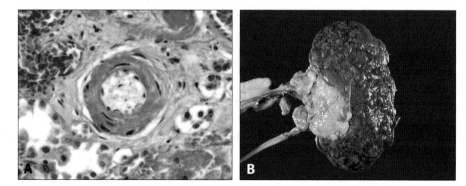

Fig. 15.13 Complications of diabetes. **A,** Hyaline arteriolosclerosis. **B,** Glomerulosclerosis.

II. HYPERCORTISOLISM (CUSHING SYNDROME)

A. Excess cortisol

B. Clinical features

    1. Muscle weakness with thin extremities—Cortisol breaks down muscle producing amino acids for gluconeogenesis.

    2. Moon facies, buffalo hump, and truncal obesity—High insulin (due to high glucose) increases storage of fat.

    3. Abdominal striae—due to impaired synthesis of collagen with thinning of skin

    4. Hypertension

    5. Osteoporosis

    6. Immune suppression

C. Diagnosis is made by increased 24-hour urine cortisol levels.

D. Causes include

    1. Exogenous corticosteroids—leads to bilateral adrenal atrophy; steroids suppress ACTH secretion (negative feedback).

    2. Primary adrenal adenoma, hyperplasia, or carcinoma—leads to atrophy of the uninvolved adrenal gland

    3. ACTH-secreting pituitary adenoma—leads to bilateral adrenal hyperplasia

    4. Paraneoplastic ACTH secretion (e.g., small cell carcinoma of the lung)—leads to bilateral adrenal hyperplasia

E. High-dose dexamethasone (cortisol analog) suppresses ACTH production by a pituitary adenoma (cortisol levels decrease), but fails to suppress ectopic ACTH production by a small cell lung carcinoma (cortisol levels remain high).

III. HYPERALDOSTERONISM (CONN SYNDROME)

A. Excess aldosterone

B. Presents as hypertension due to sodium retention, hypokalemia, and metabolic alkalosis

    1. Aldosterone increases sodium absorption and secretion of potassium and hydrogen ions (distal tubules and collecting duct).

    2. Increased absorption of sodium expands plasma volume leading to hypertension.

C. Primary hyperaldosteronism is most commonly due to sporadic adrenal hyperplasia; adrenal adenoma and adrenal carcinoma are less common causes.

    1. Characterized by high aldosterone and low renin (high blood pressure downregulates renin via negative feedback)

D. Secondary hyperaldosteronism is seen with activation of the renin-angiotensin system (e.g., renovascular hypertension or CHF).

    1. Characterized by high aldosterone and high renin

IV. CONGENITAL ADRENAL HYPERPLASIA

A. Excess sex steroids with hyperplasia of both adrenal glands

B. Inherited 21-hydroxylase deficiency is the most common cause.

    1. 21-hydroxylase is required for the production of aldosterone and corticosteroids.

    2. In enzyme deficiency, steroidogenesis is predominantly shunted toward sex steroid production (which does not require 21-hydroxylase).

    3. Deficiency of cortisol leads to increased ACTH secretion (lack of negative feedback), which results in bilateral adrenal hyperplasia.

C. Clinical features include

    1. Salt wasting with hyponatremia, hyperkalemia, and hypovolemia due to lack of aldosterone.

    2. Life-threatening hypotension due to lack of cortisol.

    3. Clitoral enlargement (females) or precocious puberty (males) due to excess androgens

V. **ADRENAL INSUFFICIENCY**

   A. Lack of adrenal hormones

   B. Acute insufficiency may arise with Waterhouse-Friderichsen syndrome.

      1. Characterized by hemorrhagic necrosis of the adrenal glands (Fig. 15.14), classically due to DIC in young children with *N meningitidis* infection

      2. Lack of cortisol exacerbates hypotension, often leading to death.

   C. Chronic insufficiency (Addison disease) is due to progressive destruction of the adrenal glands.

      1. Common causes include autoimmune destruction (most common cause in the West), TB (most common cause in the developing world), and metastatic carcinoma (e.g., arising from lung).

      2. Clinical features include hypotension, hyponatremia, hypovolemia, hyperkalemia, weakness, hyperpigmentation (increased ACTH by-products stimulate melanocytic production of pigment), vomiting, and diarrhea.

ADRENAL MEDULLA

I. **BASIC PRINCIPLES**

   A. Composed of neural crest-derived chromaffin cells

   B. Main physiologic source of catecholamines (epinephrine and norepinephrine)

II. **PHEOCHROMOCYTOMA**

   A. Tumor of chromaffin cells (Fig. 15.15)

   B. Clinical features are due to increased serum catecholamines.

      1. Episodic hypertension, headache, palpitations, tachycardia, and sweating

   C. Diagnosed by increased serum metanephrines and increased 24-hour urine metanephrines and vanillylmandelic acid

   D. Treatment is surgical excision.

      1. Catecholamines may leak into the bloodstream upon manipulation of the tumor.

      2. Phenoxybenzamine (irreversible α-blocker) is administered perioperatively to prevent a hypertensive crisis.

   E. Often follows the 'rule of 10s:' 10% bilateral, 10% familial, 10% malignant, and 10% located outside of the adrenal medulla (e.g., bladder wall or organ of Zuckerkandl at the inferior mesenteric artery root)

   F. Associated with MEN 2A and 2B, von Hippel-Lindau disease, and neurofibromatosis type 1

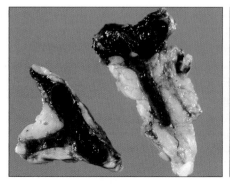

Fig. 15.14 Waterhouse-Friderichsen syndrome. (Courtesy of humpath.com)

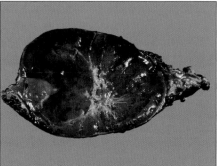

Fig. 15.15 Pheochromocytoma. (Courtesy of humpath.com)

Breast Pathology

16

INTRODUCTION

I. **BREAST**
A. Modified sweat gland embryologically derived from the skin
1. Breast tissue can develop anywhere along the milk line, which runs from the axilla to the vulva (e.g., supernumerary nipples).
B. The terminal duct lobular unit is the functional unit of the breast (Fig. 16.1); lobules make milk that drains via ducts to the nipple.
C. Lobules and ducts are lined by two layers of epithelium.
1. Luminal cell layer—inner cell layer lining the ducts and lobules; responsible for milk production in the lobules
2. Myoepithelial cell layer—outer cell layer lining ducts and lobules; contractile function propels milk towards the nipple.
D. Breast tissue is hormone sensitive.
1. Before puberty, male and female breast tissue primarily consists of large ducts under the nipple.
2. Development after menarche is primarily driven by estrogen and progesterone; lobules and small ducts form and are present in highest density in the upper outer quadrant.
3. Breast tenderness during the menstrual cycle is a common complaint, especially prior to menstruation.
4. During pregnancy, breast lobules undergo hyperplasia.
   i. Hyperplasia is driven by estrogen and progesterone produced by the corpus luteum (early first trimester), fetus, and placenta (later in pregnancy)
5. After menopause, breast tissue undergoes atrophy.
E. Galactorrhea refers to milk production outside of lactation.
1. It is not a symptom of breast cancer.
2. Causes include nipple stimulation (common physiologic cause), prolactinoma of the anterior pituitary (common pathologic cause), and drugs.

INFLAMMATORY CONDITIONS

I. **ACUTE MASTITIS**
A. Bacterial infection of the breast, usually due to *Staphylococcus aureus*
B. Associated with breast-feeding; fissures develop in the nipple providing a route of entry for microbes.
C. Presents as an erythematous breast with purulent nipple discharge; may progress to abscess formation
D. Treatment involves continued drainage (e.g., feeding) and antibiotics (e.g., dicloxacillin).

II. **PERIDUCTAL MASTITIS**
A. Inflammation of the subareolar ducts
B. Usually seen in smokers

      1.   Relative vitamin A deficiency results in squamous metaplasia of lactiferous ducts, producing duct blockage and inflammation.

   C. Clinically presents as a subareolar mass with nipple retraction

III. MAMMARY DUCT ECTASIA

   A. Inflammation with dilation (ectasia) of the subareolar ducts

      1.   Rare; classically arises in multiparous postmenopausal women

   B. Presents as a periareolar mass with green-brown nipple discharge (inflammatory debris)

      1.   Chronic inflammation with plasma cells is seen on biopsy.

IV. FAT NECROSIS

   A. Necrosis of breast fat

   B. Usually related to trauma; however, a history of trauma may not always be evident.

   C. Presents as a mass on physical exam or abnormal calcification on mammography (due to saponification)

   D. Biopsy shows necrotic fat with associated calcifications and giant cells.

BENIGN TUMORS AND FIBROCYSTIC CHANGES

I. FIBROCYSTIC CHANGE

   A. Development of fibrosis and cysts in the breast

      1.   Most common change in the premenopausal breast; thought to be hormone mediated

   B. Presents as vague irregularity of the breast tissue ('lumpy breast'), usually in the upper outer quadrant

   C. Cysts have a blue-dome appearance on gross exam.

   D. Benign, but some fibrocystic-related changes are associated with an increased risk for invasive carcinoma (increased risk applies to both breasts)

      1.   Fibrosis, cysts, and apocrine metaplasia (Fig. 16.2)—no increased risk

      2.   Ductal hyperplasia and sclerosing adenosis—2x increased risk

      3.   Atypical hyperplasia—5x increased risk

II. INTRADUCTAL PAPILLOMA

   A. Papillary growth, usually into a large duct

   B. Characterized by fibrovascular projections lined by epithelial (luminal) and myoepithelial cells

   C. Classically presents as bloody nipple discharge in a premenopausal woman

   D. Must be distinguished from papillary carcinoma, which also presents as bloody nipple discharge

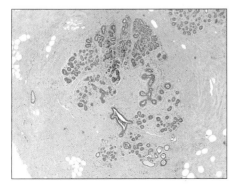

Fig. 16.1 Terminal duct lobular unit.

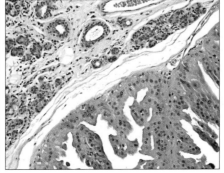

Fig. 16.2 Fibrocystic change with apocrine metaplasia.

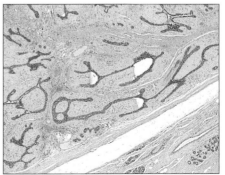

Fig. 16.3 Fibroadenoma.

1. Papillary carcinoma is characterized by fibrovascular projections lined by epithelial cells without underlying myoepithelial cells.
2. Risk of papillary carcinoma increases with age; thus, it is more commonly seen in postmenopausal women.

III. FIBROADENOMA
A. Tumor of fibrous tissue and glands (Fig. 16.3)
B. Most common benign neoplasm of the breast; usually seen in premenopausal women
C. Presents as a well-circumscribed, mobile marble-like mass
D. Estrogen sensitive—grows during pregnancy and may be painful during the menstrual cycle
E. Benign, with no increased risk of carcinoma

IV. PHYLLODES TUMOR
A. Fibroadenoma-like tumor with overgrowth of the fibrous component; characteristic 'leaf-like' projections are seen on biopsy (Fig. 16.4).
B. Most commonly seen in postmenopausal women
C. Can be malignant in some cases

BREAST CANCER

I. BASIC PRINCIPLES
A. Most common carcinoma in women by incidence (excluding skin cancer)
B. 2nd most common cause of cancer mortality in women
C. Risk factors are mostly related to estrogen exposure.
   1. Female gender
   2. Age—Cancer usually arises in postmenopausal women, with the notable exception of hereditary breast cancer.
   3. Early menarche/late menopause
   4. Obesity
   5. Atypical hyperplasia
   6. First-degree relative (mother, sister, or daughter) with breast cancer

II. DUCTAL CARCINOMA IN SITU (DCIS)
A. Malignant proliferation of cells in ducts with no invasion of the basement membrane
B. Often detected as calcification on mammography; DCIS does not usually produce a mass.
   1. Mammographic calcifications can also be associated with benign conditions such as fibrocystic changes (especially sclerosing adenosis) and fat necrosis.

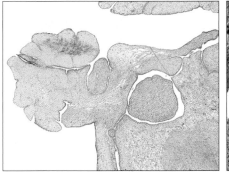
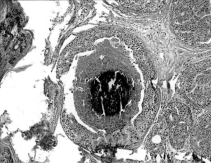

Fig. 16.4 Phyllodes tumor.   **Fig. 16.5** Ductal carcinoma in situ, comedo type.

    2. Biopsy of calcifications is often necessary to distinguish between benign and malignant conditions.

  C. Histologic subtypes are based on architecture; comedo type is characterized by high-grade cells with necrosis and dystrophic calcification in the center of ducts (Fig. 16.5).

  D. Paget disease of the breast is DCIS that extends up the ducts to involve the skin of the nipple (Fig. 16.6).

    1. Presents as nipple ulceration and erythema

    2. Paget disease of the breast is almost always associated with an underlying carcinoma.

III. INVASIVE DUCTAL CARCINOMA

  A. Invasive carcinoma that classically forms duct-like structures

  B. Most common type of invasive carcinoma in the breast, accounting for > 80% of cases

  C. Presents as a mass detected by physical exam or by mammography

    1. Clinically detected masses are usually 2 cm or greater.

    2. Mammographically detected masses are usually 1 cm or greater.

    3. Advanced tumors may result in dimpling of the skin or retraction of the nipple.

  D. Biopsy usually shows duct-like structures in a desmoplastic stroma; special subtypes of invasive ductal carcinoma include

    1. Tubular carcinoma—characterized by well-differentiated tubules that lack myoepithelial cells (Fig. 16.7A); relatively good prognosis

    2. Mucinous carcinoma—characterized by carcinoma with abundant extracellular mucin ('tumor cells floating in a mucus pool', Fig. 16.7B)

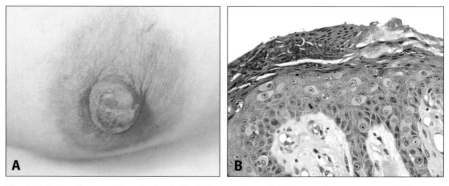

Fig. 16.6 Paget disease of the nipple. **A**, Clinical appearance. **B**, Microscopic appearance. (A, Courtesy of Jerome Taxy, MD)

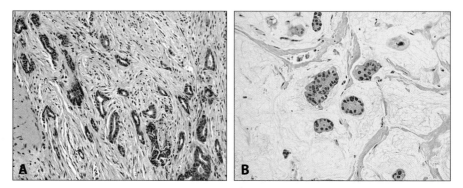

Fig. 16.7 Invasive ductal carcinoma. **A**, Tubular carcinoma. **B**, Mucinous carcinoma.

      i.   Tends to occur in older women (average age is 70 years)

      ii. Relatively good prognosis

  3. Medullary carcinoma—characterized by large, high-grade cells growing in sheets with associated lymphocytes and plasma cells

      i.   Grows as a well-circumscribed mass that can mimic fibroadenoma on mammography

      ii. Relatively good prognosis

      iii. Increased incidence in BRCA1 carriers

  4. Inflammatory carcinoma—characterized by carcinoma in dermal lymphatics (Fig. 16.8)

      i.   Presents classically as an inflamed, swollen breast (tumor cells block drainage of lymphatics) with no discrete mass; can be mistaken for acute mastitis

      ii. Poor prognosis

IV. LOBULAR CARCINOMA IN SITU (LCIS)

A. Malignant proliferation of cells in lobules with no invasion of the basement membrane

B. LCIS does not produce a mass or calcifications and is usually discovered incidentally on biopsy.

C. Characterized by dyscohesive cells lacking E-cadherin adhesion protein

D. Often multifocal and bilateral

E. Treatment is tamoxifen (to reduce the risk of subsequent carcinoma) and close follow-up; low risk of progression to invasive carcinoma

V. INVASIVE LOBULAR CARCINOMA

A. Invasive carcinoma that characteristically grows in a single-file pattern (Fig. 16.9); cells may exhibit signet-ring morphology.

  1. No duct formation due to lack of E-cadherin.

VI. PROGNOSTIC AND PREDICTIVE FACTORS

A. Prognosis in breast cancer is based on TNM staging.

  1. Metastasis is the most *important* factor, but most patients present before metastasis occurs.

  2. Spread to axillary lymph nodes is the most *useful* prognostic factor (given that metastasis is not common at presentation); sentinel lymph node biopsy is used to assess axillary lymph nodes.

B. Predictive factors predict response to treatment.

  1. Most important factors are estrogen receptor (ER), progesterone receptor (PR), and HER2/neu gene amplification (overexpression) status.

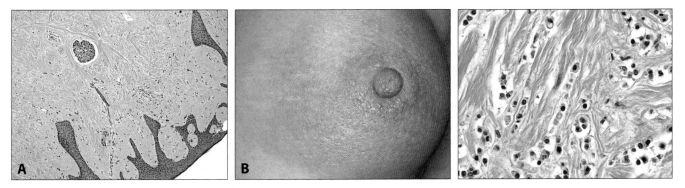

Fig. 16.8 Inflammatory carcinoma. **A,** Microscopic appearance. **B,** Clinical appearance. (B, Courtesy of Jerome Taxy, MD)　**Fig. 16.9** Invasive lobular carcinoma.

2. Presence of ER and PR is associated with response to antiestrogenic agents (e.g., tamoxifen); both receptors are located in the nucleus (Fig. 16.10).

3. HER2/neu amplification is associated with response to trastuzumab (Herceptin), a designer antibody directed against the HER2 receptor; HER2/neu is a growth factor receptor present on the cell surface (Fig. 16.11).

4. 'Triple-negative' tumors are negative for ER, PR, and HER2/neu and have a poor prognosis; African American women have an increased propensity to develop triple-negative carcinoma.

VII. HEREDITARY BREAST CANCER

A. Represents 10% of breast cancer cases

B. Clinical features that suggest hereditary breast cancer include multiple first-degree relatives with breast cancer, tumor at an early age (premenopausal), and multiple tumors in a single patient.

C. *BRCA1* and *BRCA2* mutations are the most important single gene mutations associated with hereditary breast cancer.

    1. *BRCA1* mutation is associated with breast and ovarian carcinoma.

    2. *BRCA2* mutation is associated with breast carcinoma in males.

D. Women with a genetic propensity to develop breast cancer may choose to undergo removal of both breasts (bilateral mastectomy) to decrease the risk of developing carcinoma.

    1. A small risk for cancer remains because breast tissue sometimes extends into the axilla or subcutaneous tissue of the chest wall.

VIII. MALE BREAST CANCER

A. Breast cancer is rare in males (represents 1% of all breast cancers).

B. Usually presents as a subareolar mass in older males

    1. Highest density of breast tissue in males is underneath the nipple.

    2. May produce nipple discharge

C. Most common histological subtype is invasive ductal carcinoma.

    1. Lobular carcinoma is rare (the male breast develops very few lobules).

D. Associated with *BRCA2* mutations and Klinefelter syndrome

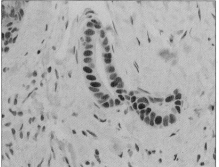

Fig. 16.10 Estrogen receptor, immunohistochemical stain.

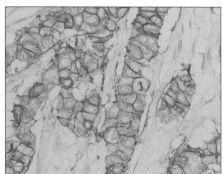

Fig. 16.11 HER2/neu amplification, immunohistochemical stain.

Central Nervous System Pathology

17

DEVELOPMENTAL ANOMALIES

I. **NEURAL TUBE DEFECTS**
   A. Arise from incomplete closure of the neural tube
      1. Neural plate invaginates early in gestation to form the neural tube, which runs along the cranial-caudal axis of the embryo.
      2. The wall of the neural tube forms central nervous system tissue, the hollow lumen forms the ventricles and spinal cord canal, and the neural crest forms the peripheral nervous system.
   B. Associated with low folate levels prior to conception
   C. Detected during prenatal care by elevated alpha-fetoprotein (AFP) levels in the amniotic fluid and maternal blood
   D. Anencephaly is absence of the skull and brain (disruption of the cranial end of the neural tube).
      1. Leads to a 'frog-like' appearance of the fetus (Fig. 17.1)
      2. Results in maternal polyhydramnios since fetal swallowing of amniotic fluid is impaired
   E. Spina bifida is failure of the posterior vertebral arch to close, resulting in a vertebral defect (disruption of the caudal end of the neural tube).
      1. Spina bifida occulta presents as a dimple or patch of hair overlying the vertebral defect.
      2. Spina bifida presents with cystic protrusion of the underlying tissue through the vertebral defect.
         i. Meningocele—protrusion of meninges
         ii. Meningomyelocele—protrusion of meninges and spinal cord

II. **CEREBRAL AQUEDUCT STENOSIS**
   A. Congenital stenosis of the channel that drains cerebrospinal fluid (CSF) from the 3rd ventricle into the 4th ventricle
   B. Leads to accumulation of CSF in the ventricular space; most common cause of hydrocephalus in newborns
      1. CSF is produced by the choroid plexus lining the ventricles.
      2. Flows from the lateral ventricles into the 3rd ventricle via the interventricular foramen of Monro
      3. Flows from the 3rd ventricle into the 4th ventricle via the cerebral aqueduct
      4. Flows from the 4th ventricle into the subarachnoid space via the foramina of Magendie and Luschka
   C. Presents with enlarging head circumference due to dilation of the ventricles (cranial suture lines are not fused)

III. **DANDY-WALKER MALFORMATION**
   A. Congenital failure of the cerebellar vermis to develop
   B. Presents as a massively dilated 4th ventricle (posterior fossa) with an absent cerebellum (Fig. 17.2); often accompanied by hydrocephalus

IV. **ARNOLD-CHIARI MALFORMATION (TYPE II)**
   A. Congenital downward displacement of cerebellar vermis and tonsils through the foramen magnum
   B. Obstruction of CSF flow commonly results in hydrocephalus.
   C. May occur in association with meningomyelocele (most cases) and syringomyelia

[handwritten: Type I no symptoms]

SPINAL CORD LESIONS

I. **SYRINGOMYELIA**
   A. Cystic degeneration of the spinal cord
   B. Arises with trauma or in association with an Arnold-Chiari malformation
   C. Usually occurs at C8-T1
      1. Presents as sensory loss of pain and temperature with sparing of fine touch and position sense in the upper extremities ("cape like" distribution)—due to involvement of the anterior white commissure of the spinothalamic tract with sparing of the dorsal column (Table 17.1)
   D. Syrinx expansion results in involvement of other spinal tracts leading to
      1. Muscle atrophy and weakness with decreased muscle tone and impaired reflexes—due to damage to lower motor neurons of the anterior horn
      2. Horner syndrome with ptosis (droopy eyelid), miosis (constricted pupil), and anhidrosis (decreased sweating)—due to disruption of the lateral horn of the hypothalamospinal tract (Table 17.1)
      [handwritten: @ T1]

[handwritten: PTA]

[handwritten: colonizes oropharynx → fever small bowel]

II. **POLIOMYELITIS**
   A. Damage to the anterior motor horn due to poliovirus infection
   B. Presents with lower motor neuron signs—flaccid paralysis with muscle atrophy, fasciculations, weakness with decreased muscle tone, impaired reflexes, and negative Babinski sign (downgoing toes)

III. **WERDNIG-HOFFMAN DISEASE**
   A. Inherited degeneration of the anterior motor horn; autosomal recessive
   B. Presents as a "floppy baby;" death occurs within a few years after birth.

IV. **AMYOTROPHIC LATERAL SCLEROSIS (ALS)**
   A. Degenerative disorder of upper and lower motor neurons of the corticospinal tract (Table 17.1)
      1. Anterior motor horn degeneration leads to lower motor neuron signs—flaccid paralysis with muscle atrophy, fasciculations, weakness with decreased muscle tone, impaired reflexes, and negative Babinski sign.

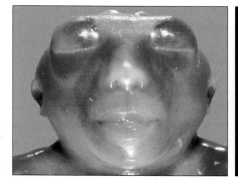

Fig. 17.1 Anencephaly. (Courtesy of humpath. com)

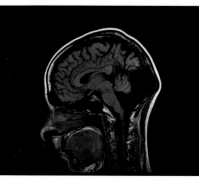

Fig. 17.2 Dandy-Walker malformation, MRI. (Courtesy of Robert Heng, MD)

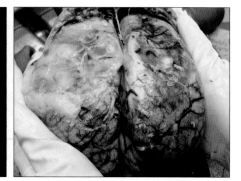

Fig. 17.3 Bacterial meningitis, gross appearance.

2. Lateral corticospinal tract degeneration leads to upper motor neuron signs—spastic paralysis with hyperreflexia, increased muscle tone, and positive Babinski sign.

B. Atrophy and weakness of hands is an early sign.

1. Lack of sensory impairment distinguishes ALS from syringomyelia.

C. Most cases are sporadic, arising in middle age adults.

1. Zinc-copper superoxide dismutase mutation (*SOD1*) is present in some familial cases; leads to free radical injury in neurons

[handwritten: SOD, $O_2^{\ominus} \rightarrow H_2O_2$]

V. FRIEDREICH ATAXIA

A. Degenerative disorder of the cerebellum and spinal cord

[handwritten: Ataxia + spinal cord tract lesions]

1. Degeneration of the cerebellum leads to ataxia.

2. Degeneration of multiple spinal cord tracts leads to loss of vibratory sense and proprioception, muscle weakness in the lower extremities, and loss of deep tendon reflexes.

B. Autosomal recessive; due to expansion of an unstable trinucleotide repeat (GAA) in the frataxin gene

1. Frataxin is essential for mitochondrial iron regulation; loss results in iron buildup with free radical damage.

C. Presents in early childhood; patients are wheelchair bound within a few years.

D. Associated with hypertrophic cardiomyopathy

MENINGITIS

I. BASIC PRINCIPLES

A. Inflammation of the leptomeninges (Fig. 17.3)

1. Meninges consist of three layers (dura, arachnoid, and pia) that lie between the brain and the skull.

2. Pia and arachnoid together are termed leptomeninges.

[handwritten: Pia against brain / dura against bone]

Table 17.1: Spinal Cord Tracts

TRACT	FIRST-ORDER NEURON	SECOND-ORDER NEURON	THIRD-ORDER NEURON
Spinothalamic (pain and temperature sensation)	Peripheral nerves to posterior horn; cell body is in dorsal root ganglion.	Arises from posterior horn, immediately crosses over in anterior white commissure, and ascends via the spinothalamic tract to thalamus	Thalamus to cortex
Dorsal column-medial lemniscus (pressure, touch, vibration, and proprioception)	Peripheral nerves to medulla via dorsal column; cell body is in dorsal root ganglion.	Arises from medulla, crosses over, and ascends via the medial lemniscus to thalamus	Thalamus to cortex
Lateral corticospinal (voluntary movement)	Pyramidal neurons in cortex descend, cross over in medullary pyramids, and synapse on the anterior motor horn of the cord (upper motor neuron).	Arises from the anterior motor horn and synapses on muscle (lower motor neuron)	(None)
Hypothalamospinal (sympathetic input of the face)	Arises from the hypothalamus and synapses on the lateral horn at T1	Arises from lateral horn at T1 and synapses on the superior cervical ganglion (sympathetic)	Superior cervical ganglion to eyelids, pupil, and skin of face

from vag get it during birth

B. Most commonly due to an infectious agent

enters via nasopharynx

   1. Group B streptococci, *E coli*, and *Listeria monocytogenes* (neonates)
   2. *N meningitidis* (children and teenagers), *Streptococcus pneumoniae* (adults and elderly), and *H influenza* (nonvaccinated infants)
   3. Coxsackievirus (children; fecal-oral transmission)
   4. Fungi (immunocompromised individuals)

C. Presents with classic triad of headache, nuchal rigidity, and fever; photophobia, vomiting, and altered mental status may also be present. *CSF w/ virus*

subarachnoid space = CSF

D. Diagnosis is made by lumbar puncture (sampling of CSF).
   1. Performed by placing a needle between L4 and L5 (level of the iliac crest). Spinal cord ends at L2, but subarachnoid space and cauda equina continue to S2.
   2. Layers crossed include skin, ligaments, epidural space, dura, and arachnoid.

E. CSF findings *don't go into pia*

normal CSF [glu] = ⅔ serum [glu]

   1. Bacterial meningitis—neutrophils with ↓ CSF glucose; gram stain and culture often identify the causative organism.
   2. Viral meningitis—lymphocytes with normal CSF glucose
   3. Fungal meningitis—lymphocytes with ↓ CSF glucose

F. Complications are usually seen with bacterial meningitis.
   1. Death—herniation secondary to cerebral edema
   2. Hydrocephalus, hearing loss, and seizures—sequelae related to fibrosis

CEREBROVASCULAR DISEASE

I. **BASIC PRINCIPLES**

A. Neurologic deficit due to cerebrovascular compromise; major cause of morbidity and mortality

B. Due to ischemia (85% of cases) or hemorrhage (15% of cases)
   1. Neurons are dependent on serum glucose as an essential energy source and are particularly susceptible to ischemia (undergo necrosis within 3–5 minutes).

II. **GLOBAL CEREBRAL ISCHEMIA**

A. Global ischemia to the brain

B. Major etiologies
   1. Low perfusion (e.g., atherosclerosis)
   2. Acute decrease in blood flow (e.g., cardiogenic shock)
   3. Chronic hypoxia (e.g., anemia)
   4. Repeated episodes of hypoglycemia (e.g., insulinoma)

C. Clinical features are based on duration and magnitude of the insult.
   1. Mild global ischemia results in transient confusion with prompt recovery.

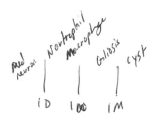

Red neuron | Neutrophil Macrophage | Gliosis | Cyst
1D   100   1M

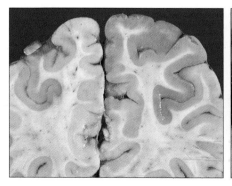

Fig. 17.4 Pale infarct, cortex. (Courtesy of Robert Wollmann, MD)

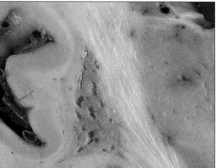

Fig. 17.5 Lacunar infarcts. (Courtesy of Robert Wollmann, MD)

2. Severe global ischemia results in diffuse necrosis; survival leads to a 'vegetative state.'
3. Moderate global ischemia leads to infarcts in watershed areas (e.g., area lying between regions fed by the anterior and middle cerebral artery) and damage to highly vulnerable regions such as
   i. Pyramidal neurons of the cerebral cortex (layers 3, 5, and 6)—leads to laminar necrosis
   ii. Pyramidal neurons of the hippocampus (temporal lobe)—important in long-term memory
   iii. Purkinje layer of the cerebellum—integrates sensory perception with motor control

III. ISCHEMIC STROKE

A. Regional ischemia to the brain that results in focal neurologic deficits lasting > 24 hours *< 24 hrs*
   1. If symptoms last < 24 hours, the event is termed a transient ischemic attack (TIA).
B. Subtypes include thrombotic, embolic, and lacunar strokes.
   1. Thrombotic stroke is due to rupture of an atherosclerotic plaque. *→ thrombi formation*
      i. Atherosclerosis usually develops at branch points (e.g., bifurcation of internal carotid and middle cerebral artery in the circle of Willis).
      ii. Results in a pale infarct at the periphery of the cortex (Fig. 17.4)
   2. Embolic stroke is due to thromboemboli.
      i. Most common source of emboli is the left side of the heart (e.g., atrial fibrillation).
      ii. Usually involves the middle cerebral artery *→ b/c thrombi is broken up & area is reperfused*
      iii. Results in a hemorrhagic infarct at the periphery of the cortex
   3. Lacunar stroke occurs secondary to hyaline arteriolosclerosis, a complication of hypertension. *↳ diabetes / benign HTN*
      i. Most commonly involves lenticulostriate vessels, resulting in small cystic areas of infarction (Fig. 17.5)
      ii. Involvement of the internal capsule leads to a pure motor stroke.
      iii. Involvement of the thalamus leads to a pure sensory stroke.
C. Ischemic stroke results in liquefactive necrosis.
   1. Eosinophilic change in the cytoplasm of neurons (red neurons, Fig. 17.6A) is an early microscopic finding (12 hours after infarction).
   2. Necrosis (24 hours), infiltration by neutrophils (days 1–3) and microglial cells (days 4–7), and gliosis (weeks 2–3) then ensue.
   3. Results in formation of a fluid-filled cystic space surrounded by gliosis (Fig. 17.6B) *↳ reactive astrocytes*

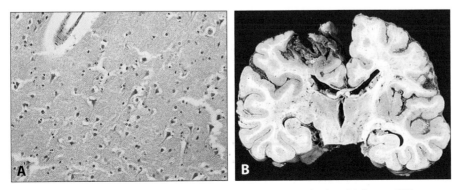

Fig. 17.6 Brain infarct. **A**, Red neurons. **B**, Cyst formation. (Courtesy of Robert Wollmann, MD)

IV. **INTRACEREBRAL HEMORRHAGE**   *hyaline arteriolosclerosis*
   A. Bleeding into brain parenchyma
   B. Classically due to rupture of Charcot-Bouchard microaneurysms of the lenticulostriate vessels
      1. Complication of hypertension; treatment of hypertension reduces incidence by half.
      2. Basal ganglia is the most common site (Fig. 17.7).
   C. Presents as severe headache, nausea, vomiting, and eventual coma

V. **SUBARACHNOID HEMORRHAGE**
   A. Bleeding into the subarachnoid space (Fig. 17.8)
   B. Presents as a sudden headache ("worst headache of my life") with nuchal rigidity
   C. Lumbar puncture shows xanthochromia (yellow hue due to bilirubin breakdown).
   D. Most frequently (85%) due to rupture of a berry aneurysm; other causes include AV malformations and an anticoagulated state.
      1. Berry aneurysms are thin-walled saccular outpouchings that lack a media layer (Fig. 17.9), increasing the risk for rupture.
      2. Most frequently located in the anterior circle of Willis at branch points of the anterior communicating artery
      3. Associated with Marfan syndrome and autosomal dominant polycystic kidney disease   *Adult*

TRAUMA

dura is tightly attached to skull

I. **EPIDURAL HEMATOMA**
   A. Collection of blood between the dura and the skull
   B. Classically due to fracture of the temporal bone with rupture of the middle meningeal artery; bleeding separates the dura from the skull.
      1. Lens-shaped lesion on CT
      2. Lucid interval may precede neurologic signs.
   C. Herniation is a lethal complication.

II. **SUBDURAL HEMATOMA**
   A. Collection of blood underneath the dura; blood covers the surface of the brain (Fig. 17.10).
   B. Due to tearing of bridging veins that lie between the dura and arachnoid; usually arises with trauma
      1. Crescent-shaped lesion on CT
      2. Presents with progressive neurologic signs

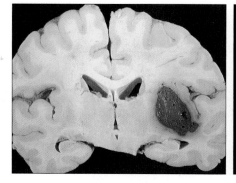
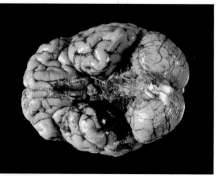

Fig. 17.7 Intracerebral hemorrhage, basal ganglia. (Courtesy of Robert Wollmann, MD)

Fig. 17.8 Subarachnoid hemorrhage. (Courtesy of Jerome Taxy, MD)

3. Increased rate of occurrence in the elderly due to age-related cerebral atrophy, which stretches the veins

C. Herniation is a lethal complication.

III. HERNIATION

A. Displacement of brain tissue due to mass effect or increased intracranial pressure

B. Tonsillar herniation involves displacement of the cerebellar tonsils into the foramen magnum.
1. Compression of the brain stem leads to cardiopulmonary arrest.

C. Subfalcine herniation involves displacement of the cingulate gyrus under the falx cerebri.
1. Compression of the anterior cerebral artery leads to infarction.

D. Uncal herniation involves displacement of the temporal lobe uncus under the tentorium cerebelli.
1. Compression of cranial nerve III (oculomotor) leads to the eye moving "down and out" and a dilated pupil.
2. Compression of posterior cerebral artery leads to infarction of occipital lobe (contralateral homonymous hemianopsia).
3. Rupture of the paramedian artery leads to Duret (brainstem) hemorrhage.

DEMYELINATING DISORDERS

I. BASIC PRINCIPLES

A. Myelin insulates axons, improving the speed and efficiency of conduction.
1. Oligodendrocytes myelinate the central nervous system.
2. Schwann cells myelinate the peripheral nervous system.

B. Demyelinating disorders are characterized by destruction of myelin or oligodendrocytes; axons are generally preserved.

II. LEUKODYSTROPHIES

A. Inherited mutations in enzymes necessary for production or maintenance of myelin

B. Metachromatic leukodystrophy is due to a deficiency of arylsulfatase (autosomal recessive); most common leukodystrophy   *can't degrade myelin*
1. Sulfatides cannot be degraded and accumulate in the lysosomes of oligodendrocytes (lysosomal storage disease).

C. Krabbe disease is due to a deficiency of galactocerebrosidase (autosomal recessive).
1. Galactocerebroside accumulates in macrophages.

D. Adrenoleukodystrophy is due to impaired addition of coenzyme A to long-chain fatty acids (X-linked defect).

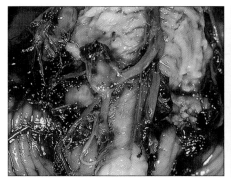

Fig. 17.9 Berry aneurysm. (Courtesy of Jerome Taxy, MD)

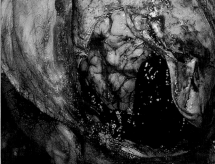

Fig. 17.10 Subdural hematoma. (Courtesy of Robert Wollmann, MD)

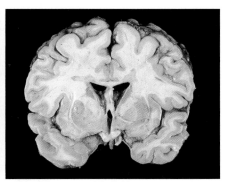

Fig. 17.11 Gray plaque, multiple sclerosis. (Courtesy of Peter Pytel, MD)

1. Accumulation of fatty acids damages adrenal glands and white matter of the brain.

III. **MULTIPLE SCLEROSIS**
   A. Autoimmune destruction of CNS myelin and oligodendrocytes
      1. Most common chronic CNS disease of young adults (20–30 years of age); more commonly seen in women
      2. Associated with HLA-DR2
      3. More commonly seen in regions away from the equator
   B. Presents with relapsing neurologic deficits with periods of remission (multiple lesions in time and space). Clinical features include
      1. Blurred vision in one eye (optic nerve)
      2. Vertigo and scanning speech mimicking alcohol intoxication (brainstem)
      3. Internuclear ophthalmoplegia (medial longitudinal fasciculus)
      4. Hemiparesis or unilateral loss of sensation (cerebral white matter, usually periventricular)
      5. Lower extremity loss of sensation or weakness (spinal cord)
      6. Bowel, bladder, and sexual dysfunction (autonomic nervous system)
   C. Diagnosis is made by MRI and lumbar puncture.
      1. MRI reveals plaques (areas of white matter demyelination).
      2. Lumbar puncture shows increased lymphocytes, increased immunoglobulins with oligoclonal IgG bands on high resolution electrophoresis, and myelin basic protein.
   D. Gross examination shows gray-appearing plaques in the white matter (Fig. 17.11).
   E. Treatment of acute attacks includes high-dose steroids.
      1. Long-term treatment with interferon beta slows progression of disease.

IV. **SUBACUTE SCLEROSING PANENCEPHALITIS**
   A. Progressive, debilitating encephalitis leading to death
   B. Due to slowly progressing, persistent infection of the brain by measles virus.
      1. Infection occurs in infancy; neurologic signs arise years later (during childhood).
   C. Characterized by viral inclusions within neurons (gray matter) and oligodendrocytes (white matter)

V. **PROGRESSIVE MULTIFOCAL LEUKOENCEPHALOPATHY**
   A. JC virus infection of oligodendrocytes (white matter)
      1. Immunosuppression (e.g., AIDS or leukemia) leads to reactivation of the latent virus.
   B. Presents with rapidly progressive neurologic signs (visual loss, weakness, dementia) leading to death

VI. **CENTRAL PONTINE MYELINOLYSIS**
   A. Focal demyelination of the pons (anterior brain stem)
   B. Due to rapid intravenous correction of hyponatremia
      1. Occurs in severely malnourished patients (e.g., alcoholics and patients with liver disease)
   C. Classically presents as acute bilateral paralysis ("locked in" syndrome)

DEMENTIA AND DEGENERATIVE DISORDERS

I. **BASIC PRINCIPLES**
   A. Characterized by loss of neurons within the gray matter; often due to accumulation of protein which damages neurons

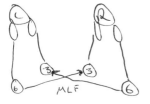

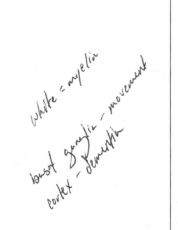

B. Degeneration of the cortex leads to dementia.

C. Degeneration of the brainstem and basal ganglia leads to movement disorders.

II. ALZHEIMER DISEASE (AD)

A. Degenerative disease of cortex; most common cause of dementia

B. Clinical features

1. Slow-onset memory loss (begins with short-term memory loss and progresses to long-term memory loss) and progressive disorientation

2. Loss of learned motor skills and language

3. Changes in behavior and personality

4. Patients become mute and bedridden; infection is a common cause of death.

5. Focal neurologic deficits are not seen in early disease.

C. Most cases (95%) are sporadic and seen in the elderly.

1. Risk increases with age (doubles every 5 years after the age of 60).

2. ε4 allele of apolipoprotein E (*APOE*) is associated with increased risk, ε2 allele with decreased risk.

D. Early-onset AD is seen in

1. Familial cases—associated with presenilin 1 and presenilin 2 mutations

2. Down syndrome—commonly occurs by 40 years of age *b/c APP is on chrom 21*

E. Morphologic features include

1. Cerebral atrophy with narrowing of the gyri, widening of the sulci, and dilation of the ventricles (Fig. 17.12A)   *hydrocephalus ex vacuo*

2. Neuritic plaques—extracellular core comprised of Aβ amyloid with entangled neuritic processes (Fig. 17.12B)   *Amyloid is always extracellular*

   i. Aβ amyloid is derived from amyloid precursor protein (APP), which is coded on chromosome 21. APP normally undergoes alpha cleavage; beta cleavage results in Aβ amyloid.

   ii. Amyloid may also deposit around vessels, increasing the risk of hemorrhage.

3. Neurofibrillary tangles—intracellular aggregates of fibers composed of hyperphosphorylated tau protein (Fig. 17.12C)

   i. Tau is a microtubule-associated protein.

4. Loss of cholinergic neurons in the nucleus basalis of Meynert *= ↓ ACh*

F. Diagnosis is made by clinical and pathological correlation.

1. Presumptive diagnosis is made clinically after excluding other causes.

2. Confirmed by histology at autopsy (when possible)

III. VASCULAR DEMENTIA

A. Multifocal infarction and injury due to hypertension, atherosclerosis, or vasculitis

B. 2nd most common cause of dementia

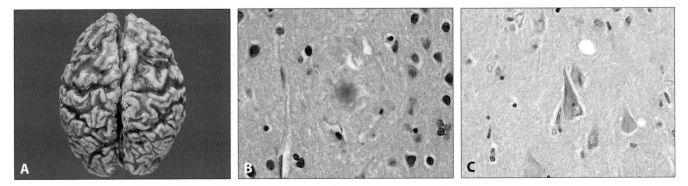

Fig. 17.12 Alzheimer disease. **A**, Cerebral atrophy. **B**, Neuritic plaque. **C**, Neurofibrillary tangle. (A, Courtesy of Jerome Taxy, MD. B and C, Courtesy of Peter Pytel, MD)

IV. **PICK DISEASE**
   A. Degenerative disease of the frontal and temporal cortex; spares the parietal and occipital lobes
   B. Characterized by round aggregates of tau protein (Pick bodies) in neurons of the cortex
   C. Behavioral and language symptoms arise early; eventually progresses to dementia

V. **PARKINSON DISEASE**
   A. Degenerative loss of dopaminergic neurons in the substantia nigra of the basal ganglia (Fig. 17.13A,B) $D_1 + D_2$
      1. Nigrostriatal pathway of basal ganglia uses dopamine to initiate movement.
   B. Common disorder related to aging; seen in 2% of older adults
   C. Unknown etiology; historically, rare cases were related to MPTP exposure (a contaminant in illicit drugs).
   D. Clinical features ('TRAP')
      1. Tremor—pill rolling tremor at rest; disappears with movement
      2. Rigidity—cogwheel rigidity in the extremities
      3. Akinesia/bradykinesia—slowing of voluntary movement; expressionless face
      4. Postural instability and shuffling gait
   E. Histology reveals loss of pigmented neurons in the substantia nigra and round, eosinophilic inclusions of α-synuclein (Lewy bodies, Fig. 17.13C) in affected neurons.
   F. Dementia is a common feature of late disease.
      1. Early-onset dementia is suggestive of Lewy body dementia, which is characterized by dementia, hallucinations and parkinsonian features; histology reveals cortical Lewy bodies.

VI. **HUNTINGTON DISEASE**
   A. Degeneration of GABAergic neurons in the caudate nucleus of the basal ganglia (Fig. 17.14)   *you lose inhibition of movement pathways so you get random movement*
      1. Autosomal dominant disorder (chromosome 4) characterized by expanded trinucleotide repeats (CAG) in the huntingtin gene
      2. Further expansion of repeats during spermatogenesis leads to anticipation.
   B. Presents with chorea that can progress to dementia and depression; average age at presentation is 40 years.   *→ rapid involuntary contraction of muscle*
   C. Suicide is a common cause of death.

Striatum = caudate + putamen

VII. **NORMAL PRESSURE HYDROCEPHALUS**
   A. Increased CSF resulting in dilated ventricles
   B. Can cause dementia in adults; usually idiopathic

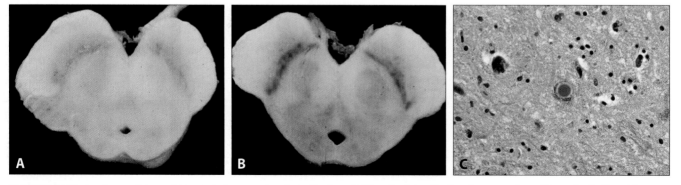

Fig. 17.13 Parkinson disease. **A**, Loss of pigmented neurons in substantia nigra. **B**, Normal substantia nigra for comparison. **C**, Lewy body. (A and B, Courtesy of Robert Wollmann, MD)

C. Presents as triad of urinary incontinence, gait instability, and dementia ("wet, wobbly, and wacky") *stretching of corona radiata*

D. Lumbar puncture improves symptoms; treatment is ventriculoperitoneal shunting.

Arachnoid granulations

VIII. **SPONGIFORM ENCEPHALOPATHY**

A. Degenerative disease due to prion protein

    1. Prion protein is normally expressed in CNS neurons in an α-helical configuration (PrP^c).

B. Disease arises with conversion to a β-pleated conformation (PrP^{sc}).

    1. Conversion can be sporadic, inherited (familial forms of disease), or transmitted.

C. Pathologic protein is not degradable and converts normal protein into the pathologic form, resulting in a vicious cycle.

    1. Damage to neurons and glial cells is characterized by intracellular vacuoles (spongy degeneration, Fig. 17.15).

D. Creutzfeldt-Jakob disease (CJD) is the most common spongiform encephalopathy.

    1. Usually sporadic; rarely can arise due to exposure to prion-infected human tissue (e.g., human growth hormone or corneal transplant)

    2. Presents as rapidly progressive dementia associated with ataxia (cerebellar involvement) and startle myoclonus

        i. Periodic sharp waves are seen on EEG.

        ii. Results in death, usually in < 1 year

    3. Variant CJD is a special form of disease that is related to exposure to bovine spongiform encephalopathy ('mad cow').

E. Familial fatal insomnia is an inherited form of prion disease characterized by severe insomnia and an exaggerated startle response.

CNS TUMORS

I. **BASIC PRINCIPLES**

A. Can be metastatic (50%) or primary (50%)

B. Metastatic tumors characteristically present as multiple, well-circumscribed lesions at the gray-white junction.

    1. Lung, breast, and kidney are common sources.

C. Primary tumors are classified according to cell type of origin (e.g., astrocytes, meningothelial cells, ependymal cells, oligodendrocytes, or neuroectoderm).

D. In adults, primary tumors are usually supratentorial.

    1. Most common tumors in adults are glioblastoma multiforme, meningioma, and schwannoma.

E. In children, primary tumors are usually infratentorial.

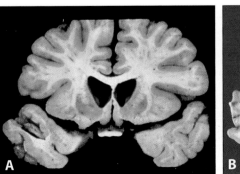
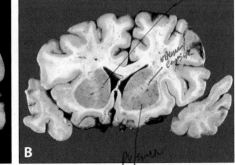
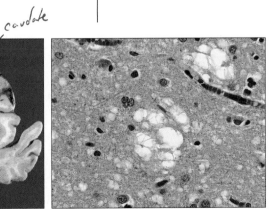

Fig. 17.14 Huntington disease. **A**, Degeneration of caudate nucleus. **B**, Normal caudate nucleus for comparison. (Courtesy of Peter Pytel, MD)

Fig. 17.15 Spongiform encephalopathy. (Courtesy of Peter Pytel, MD)

1. Most common tumors in children are pilocytic astrocytoma, ependymoma, and medulloblastoma.

F. Primary malignant CNS tumors are locally destructive, but rarely metastasize.

II. GLIOBLASTOMA MULTIFORME (GBM)

A. Malignant, high-grade tumor of astrocytes

B. Most common primary malignant CNS tumor in adults

C. Usually arises in the cerebral hemisphere; characteristically crosses the corpus callosum ('butterfly' lesion, Fig. 17.16A)

D. Characterized by regions of necrosis surrounded by tumor cells (pseudopalisading, Fig. 17.16B) and endothelial cell proliferation; tumor cells are GFAP positive.

E. Poor prognosis

III. MENINGIOMA

A. Benign tumor of arachnoid cells

B. Most common benign CNS tumor in adults
   1. More commonly seen in women; rare in children

C. May present as seizures; tumor compresses, but does not invade, the cortex.

D. Imaging reveals a round mass attached to the dura.

E. Histology shows a whorled pattern (Fig. 17.17); psammoma bodies may be present.

IV. SCHWANNOMA

A. Benign tumor of Schwann cells

B. Involves cranial or spinal nerves; within the cranium, most frequently involves cranial nerve VIII at the cerebellopontine angle (presents as loss of hearing and tinnitus)

C. Tumor cells are S-100 positive.

D. Bilateral tumors are seen in neurofibromatosis type 2.

V. OLIGODENDROGLIOMA

A. Malignant tumor of oligodendrocytes

B. Imaging reveals a calcified tumor in the white matter, usually involving the frontal lobe; may present with seizures

C. 'Fried-egg' appearance of cells on biopsy (Fig. 17.18)

VI. PILOCYTIC ASTROCYTOMA

A. Benign tumor of astrocytes

B. Most common CNS tumor in children; usually arises in the cerebellum

C. Imaging reveals a cystic lesion with a mural nodule (Fig. 17.19A).

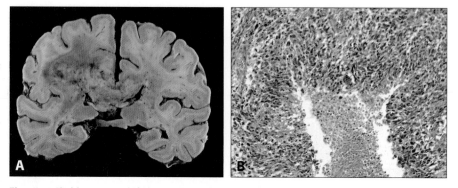

Fig. 17.16 Glioblastoma multiforme. **A,** 'Butterfly' lesion. **B,** Pseudopalisading. (Courtesy of Peter Pytel, MD)

D. Biopsy shows Rosenthal fibers (thick eosinophilic processes of astrocytes, Fig. 17.19B) and eosinophilic granular bodies; tumor cells are GFAP positive.

VII. MEDULLOBLASTOMA
A. Malignant tumor derived from the granular cells of the cerebellum (neuroectoderm)
B. Usually arises in children
C. Histology reveals small, round blue cells; Homer-Wright rosettes may be present.
D. Poor prognosis; tumor grows rapidly and spreads via CSF.
   1. Metastasis to the cauda equina is termed 'drop metastasis.'

VIII. EPENDYMOMA
A. Malignant tumor of ependymal cells; usually seen in children
B. Most commonly arises in the 4th ventricle; may present with hydrocephalus
C. Perivascular pseudorosettes are a characteristic finding on biopsy (Fig. 17.20).

IX. CRANIOPHARYNGIOMA
A. Tumor that arises from epithelial remnants of Rathke's pouch
B. Presents as a supratentorial mass in a child or young adult; may compress the optic chiasm leading to bitemporal hemianopsia
C. Calcifications are commonly seen on imaging (derived from "tooth-like" tissue).
D. Benign, but tends to recur after resection

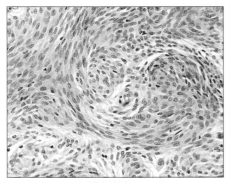

Fig. 17.17 Meningioma.

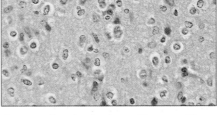

Fig. 17.18 Oligodendroglioma. (Courtesy of Peter Pytel, MD)

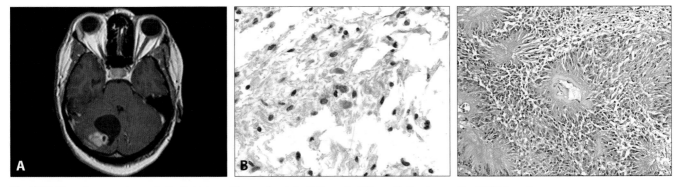

Fig. 17.19 Pilocytic astrocytoma. **A**, Cystic lesion with mural nodule. **B**, Rosenthal fibers. (A, Courtesy of Peter Pytel, MD)

Fig. 17.20 Ependymoma.

Musculoskeletal Pathology

18

SKELETAL SYSTEM

I. **ACHONDROPLASIA**
   A. Impaired cartilage proliferation in the growth plate; common cause of dwarfism
   B. Due to an activating mutation in fibroblast growth factor receptor 3 (*FGFR3*); autosomal dominant
      1. Overexpression of *FGFR3* inhibits growth.
      2. Most mutations are sporadic and related to increased paternal age.
   C. Clinical features
      1. Short extremities with normal-sized head and chest—due to poor endochondral bone formation; intramembranous bone formation is not affected.
         i. Endochondral bone formation is characterized by formation of a cartilage matrix, which is then replaced by bone; it is the mechanism by which long bones grow.
         ii. Intramembranous bone formation is characterized by formation of bone without a preexisting cartilage matrix; it is the mechanism by which flat bones (e.g., skull and rib cage) develop.
   D. Mental function, life span, and fertility are not affected.

II. **OSTEOGENESIS IMPERFECTA**
   A. Congenital defect of bone formation resulting in structurally weak bone
   B. Most commonly due to an autosomal dominant defect in collagen type I synthesis
   C. Clinical features
      1. Multiple fractures of bone (can mimic child abuse, but bruising is absent)
      2. Blue sclera—Thinning of scleral collagen reveals underlying choroidal veins.
      3. Hearing loss—Bones of the middle ear easily fracture.

III. **OSTEOPETROSIS**
   A. Inherited defect of bone resorption resulting in abnormally thick, heavy bone that fractures easily
   B. Due to poor osteoclast function
   C. Multiple genetic variants exist; carbonic anhydrase II mutation leads to loss of the acidic microenvironment required for bone resorption.
   D. Clinical features include
      1. Bone fractures
      2. Anemia, thrombocytopenia, and leukopenia with extramedullary hematopoiesis—due to bony replacement of the marrow (myelophthisic process, Fig. 18.1)
      3. Vision and hearing impairment—due to impingement on cranial nerves
      4. Hydrocephalus—due to narrowing of the foramen magnum
      5. Renal tubular acidosis—seen with carbonic anhydrase II mutation
         i. Lack of carbonic anhydrase results in decreased tubular reabsorption of HCO_3^-, leading to metabolic acidosis.
   E. Treatment is bone marrow transplant; osteoclasts are derived from monocytes.

IV. **RICKETS/OSTEOMALACIA**
  A. Defective mineralization of osteoid
    1. Osteoblasts normally produce osteoid, which is then mineralized with calcium and phosphate to form bone.
  B. Due to low levels of vitamin D, which results in low serum calcium and phosphate
    1. Vitamin D is normally derived from the skin upon exposure to sunlight (85%) and from the diet (15%).
    2. Activation requires 25-hydroxylation by the liver followed by 1-alpha-hydroxylation by the proximal tubule cells of the kidney.
    3. Active vitamin D raises serum calcium and phosphate by acting on
       i. Intestine—increases absorption of calcium and phosphate
       ii. Kidney—increases reabsorption of calcium and phosphate
       iii. Bone—increases resorption of calcium and phosphate
    4. Vitamin D deficiency is seen with decreased sun exposure (e.g., northern latitudes), poor diet, malabsorption, liver failure, and renal failure.
  C. Rickets is due to low vitamin D in children, resulting in abnormal bone mineralization.
    1. Most commonly arises in children < 1 year of age; presents with
       i. Pigeon-breast deformity—inward bending of the ribs with anterior protrusion of the sternum
       ii. Frontal bossing (enlarged forehead)—due to osteoid deposition on the skull
       iii. Rachitic rosary—due to osteoid deposition at the costochondral junction
       iv. Bowing of the legs may be seen in ambulating children.
  D. Osteomalacia is due to low vitamin D in adults.
    1. Inadequate mineralization results in weak bone with an increased risk for fracture.
    2. Laboratory findings include ↓ serum calcium, ↓ serum phosphate, ↑ PTH, and ↑ alkaline phosphatase.

V. **OSTEOPOROSIS**
  A. Reduction in trabecular bone mass
  B. Results in porous bone with an increased risk for fracture
  C. Risk of osteoporosis is based on peak bone mass (attained in early adulthood) and rate of bone loss that follows thereafter.
    1. Peak bone mass is achieved by 30 years of age and is based on (1) genetics (e.g., vitamin D receptor variants), (2) diet, and (3) exercise.
    2. Thereafter, slightly less than 1% of bone mass is lost each year; bone mass is lost more quickly with lack of weight-bearing exercise (e.g., space travel), poor diet, or decreased estrogen (e.g., menopause).
  D. Most common forms of osteoporosis are senile and postmenopausal.

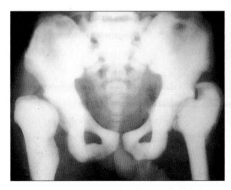

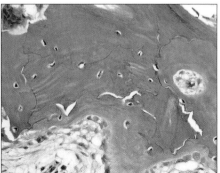

Fig. 18.1 Osteopetrosis. (Published with permission from LearningRadiology.com)

Fig. 18.2 Paget disease of bone.

E. Clinical features
    1. Bone pain and fractures in weight-bearing areas such as the vertebrae (leads to loss of height and kyphosis), hip, and distal radius
    2. Bone density is measured using a DEXA scan.
    3. Serum calcium, phosphate, PTH, and alkaline phosphatase are normal; labs help to exclude osteomalacia (which has a similar clinical presentation).
F. Treatment includes
    1. Exercise, vitamin D, and calcium—limit bone loss
    2. Bisphosphonates—induce apoptosis of osteoclasts
    3. Estrogen replacement therapy is debated (currently not recommended).
    4. Glucocorticoids are contraindicated (worsen osteoporosis).

VI. **PAGET DISEASE OF BONE**
    A. Imbalance between osteoclast and osteoblast function
        1. Usually seen in late adulthood (average age > 60 years)
    B. Etiology is unknown; possibly viral
    C. Localized process involving one or more bones; does not involve the entire skeleton
    D. Three distinct stages are (1) osteoclastic, (2) mixed osteoblastic-osteoclastic, and (3) osteoblastic.
        1. End result is thick, sclerotic bone that fractures easily.
        2. Biopsy reveals a mosaic pattern of lamellar bone (Fig. 18.2).
    E. Clinical features
        1. Bone pain—due to microfractures
        2. Increasing hat size—Skull is commonly affected.
        3. Hearing loss—impingement on cranial nerve
        4. Lion-like facies—involvement of craniofacial bones
        5. Isolated elevated alkaline phosphatase—most common cause of isolated elevated alkaline phosphatase in patients > 40 years old
    F. Treatment includes
        1. Calcitonin—inhibits osteoclast function
        2. Bisphosphonates—induces apoptosis of osteoclasts
    G. Complications include
        1. High-output cardiac failure—due to formation of AV shunts in bone
        2. Osteosarcoma

VII. **OSTEOMYELITIS**
    A. Infection of marrow and bone
        1. Usually occurs in children
    B. Most commonly bacterial; arises via hematogenous spread
        1. Transient bacteremia (children) seeds metaphysis.
        2. Open-wound bacteremia (adults) seeds epiphysis.
    C. Causes include
        1. *Staphylococcus aureus*—most common cause (90% of cases)
        2. *N gonorrhoeae*—sexually active young adults
        3. *Salmonella*—sickle cell disease
        4. *Pseudomonas*—diabetics or IV drug abusers
        5. *Pasteurella*—associated with cat or dog bite/scratches
        6. *Mycobacterium tuberculosis*—usually involves vertebrae (Pott disease)
    D. Clinical features
        1. Bone pain with systemic signs of infection (e.g., fever and leukocytosis)
        2. Lytic focus (abscess) surrounded by sclerosis of bone on x-ray; lytic focus is called sequestrum, and sclerosis is called involucrum.
    E. Diagnosis is made by blood culture.

VIII. **AVASCULAR (ASEPTIC) NECROSIS**
   A. Ischemic necrosis of bone and bone marrow
   B. Causes include trauma or fracture (most common), steroids, sickle cell anemia, and caisson disease.
   C. Osteoarthritis and fracture are major complications.

BONE TUMORS

I. **OSTEOMA**
   A. Benign tumor of bone
   B. Most commonly arises on the surface of facial bones
   C. Associated with Gardner syndrome
      ↳ fibromitosis + osteome + familial adenomatous polyposis in retroperitoneum

II. **OSTEOID OSTEOMA**
   A. Benign tumor of osteoblasts (that produce osteoid) surrounded by a rim of reactive bone   *↳mineralized by Ca + PO₄*
   B. Occurs in young adults < 25 years of age (more common in males)
   C. Arises in cortex of long bones (e.g., femur)   *cortex = surface of bone medulla = middle*
   D. Presents as bone pain that resolves with aspirin
   E. Imaging reveals a bony mass (< 2 cm) with a radiolucent core (osteoid).
   F. Osteoblastoma is similar to osteoid osteoma but is larger (> 2 cm), arises in vertebrae, and presents as bone pain that does not respond to aspirin.

III. **OSTEOCHONDROMA**
   A. Tumor of bone with an overlying cartilage cap (Fig. 18.3); most common benign tumor of bone
   B. Arises from a lateral projection of the growth plate (metaphysis); bone is continuous with the marrow space.   *that grows out of bone*
   C. Overlying cartilage can transform (rarely) to chondrosarcoma.

IV. **OSTEOSARCOMA**
   A. Malignant proliferation of osteoblasts
   B. Peak incidence is seen in teenagers; less commonly seen in the elderly
      1. Risk factors include familial retinoblastoma, Paget disease, and radiation exposure.
      2. Arises in the metaphysis of long bones, usually the distal femur or proximal tibia (region of the knee)
   C. Presents as a pathologic fracture or bone pain with swelling
   D. Imaging reveals a destructive mass with a 'sunburst' appearance and lifting of the periosteum (Codman triangle, Fig. 18.4A).

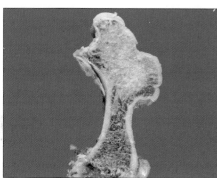

Fig. 18.3 Osteochondroma. (Courtesy of humpath.com)

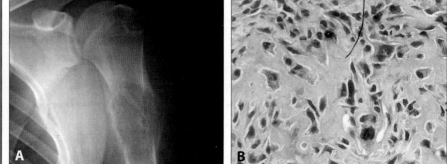

osteoid

Fig. 18.4 Osteosarcoma. **A**, X-ray. **B**, Microscopic appearance. (A, Courtesy of Bulent Celasun, MD)

E. Biopsy reveals pleomorphic cells that produce osteoid (Fig. 18.4B).

V. GIANT CELL TUMOR
A. Tumor comprised of multinucleated giant cells and stromal cells
B. Occurs in young adults
C. Arises in the epiphysis of long bones, usually the distal femur or proximal tibia (region of the knee)   *only tumor in epiphysis*
D. 'Soap-bubble' appearance on x-ray
E. Locally aggressive tumor; may recur

VI. EWING SARCOMA
A. Malignant proliferation of poorly-differentiated cells derived from neuroectoderm.
B. Arises in the diaphysis of long bones; usually in male children (< 15 years of age)
C. 'Onion-skin' appearance on x-ray
D. Biopsy reveals small, round blue cells that resemble lymphocytes (Fig. 18.5).
  1. Can be confused with lymphoma or chronic osteomyelitis
  2. (11;22) translocation is characteristic.
E. Often presents with metastasis; responsive to chemotherapy

VII. CHONDROMA
cartilage tumors = medulla
A. Benign tumor of cartilage
B. Usually arises in the medulla of small bones of the hands and feet (Fig. 18.6)
   (Periphery)

VIII. CHONDROSARCOMA
A. Malignant cartilage-forming tumor
B. Arises in medulla of the pelvis or central skeleton

IX. METASTATIC TUMORS
A. More common than primary tumors
B. Usually result in osteolytic (punched-out) lesions
  1. Prostatic carcinoma classically produces osteoblastic lesions.

JOINT

I. BASIC PRINCIPLES
A. Connection between two bones
B. Solid joints are tightly connected to provide structural strength (e.g., cranial sutures).
C. Synovial joints have a joint space to allow for motion.
  1. Articular surface of adjoining bones is made of hyaline cartilage (type II collagen) that is surrounded by a joint capsule.

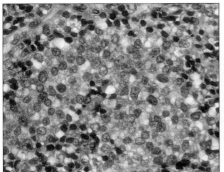

Fig. 18.5 Ewing sarcoma.

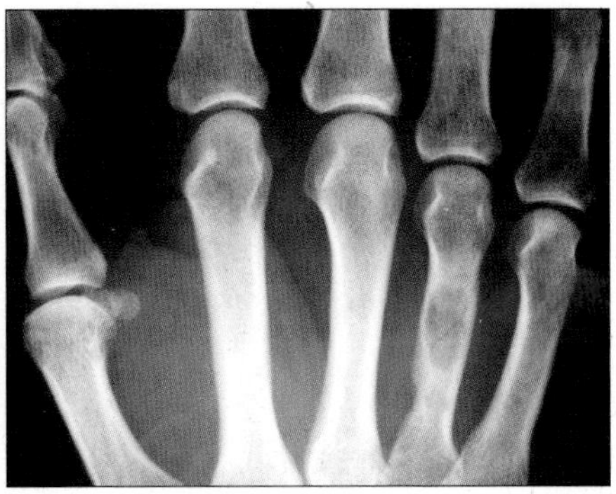

Fig. 18.6 Chondroma. (Published with permission from LearningRadiology.com)

2. Synovium lining the joint capsule secretes fluid rich in hyaluronic acid to lubricate the joint and facilitate smooth motion.

II. DEGENERATIVE JOINT DISEASE (OSTEOARTHRITIS)

A. Progressive degeneration of articular cartilage; most common type of arthritis

B. Most often due to 'wear and tear'

C. Major risk factor is age (common after 60 years); additional risk factors include obesity and trauma.

D. Affects a limited number of joints (oligoarticular); hips, lower lumbar spine, knees, and the distal interphalangeal joints (DIP) and proximal interphalangeal joints (PIP) of fingers are common sites.

E. Classic presentation is joint stiffness in the morning that worsens during the day.

F. Pathologic features include

1. Disruption of the cartilage that lines the articular surface (Fig. 18.7); fragments of cartilage floating in the joint space are called 'joint mice.'

2. Eburnation of the subchondral bone

3. Osteophyte formation (reactive bony outgrowths); classically arises in the DIP (Heberden nodes) and PIP (Bouchard nodes) joints of the fingers

III. RHEUMATOID ARTHRITIS

A. Chronic, systemic autoimmune disease

1. Classically arises in women of late childbearing age

2. Associated with HLA-DR4

B. Characterized by involvement of joints

Pull joint → fibroblast → myofibroblast ↑

1. Hallmark is synovitis leading to formation of a pannus (inflamed granulation tissue). *(→inflammation of synovium*

2. Leads to destruction of cartilage and ankylosis (fusion) of the joint

C. Clinical features

1. Arthritis with morning stiffness that improves with activity.

   i. Symmetric involvement of PIP joints of the fingers (swan-neck deformity), wrists (radial deviation), elbows, ankles, and knees is characteristic (Fig. 18.8); DIP is usually spared (unlike osteoarthritis).

   ii. Joint-space narrowing, loss of cartilage, and osteopenia are seen on x-ray.

2. Fever, malaise, weight loss, and myalgias

3. Rheumatoid nodules—central zone of necrosis surrounded by epithelioid histiocytes; arise in skin and visceral organs

4. Vasculitis—Multiple organs may be involved.

5. Baker cyst—swelling of bursa behind the knee

6. Pleural effusions, lymphadenopathy, and interstitial lung fibrosis

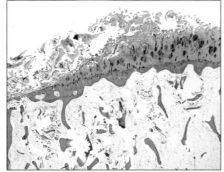

Fig. 18.7 Degenerative joint disease.

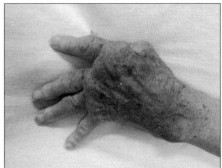

Fig. 18.8 Rheumatoid arthritis. (Courtesy of James Heilman, MD, Wikipedia)

D. Laboratory findings
   1. IgM autoantibody against Fc portion of IgG (rheumatoid factor); marker of tissue damage and disease activity
   2. Neutrophils and high protein in synovial fluid
E. Complications include anemia of chronic disease and secondary amyloidosis.

[handwritten: →Acute Phase Reactants]
[handwritten: ↳ b/c hepcidin ↳ Fe sequestration ↳ Amyloid associated protein]

IV. SERONEGATIVE SPONDYLOARTHROPATHIES
A. Group of joint disorders characterized by
   1. Lack of rheumatoid factor
   2. Axial skeleton involvement
   3. HLA-B27 association
B. Ankylosing spondyloarthritis involves the sacroiliac joints and spine.
   1. Arises in young adults, most often male
   2. Presents with low back pain; involvement of vertebral bodies eventually arises, leading to fusion of the vertebrae ('bamboo spine').
   3. Extra-articular manifestations include uveitis and aortitis (leading to aortic regurgitation).
C. Reiter syndrome is characterized by the triad of arthritis, urethritis, and conjunctivitis.
   1. Arises in young adults (usually males) weeks after a GI or *Chlamydia trachomatis* infection
D. Psoriatic arthritis is seen in 10% of cases of psoriasis.
   1. Involves axial and peripheral joints; DIP joints of the hands and feet are most commonly affected, leading to "sausage" fingers or toes.

V. INFECTIOUS ARTHRITIS
A. Arthritis due to an infectious agent, usually bacterial
B. Causes include
   1. *N gonorrhoeae*—young adults; most common cause
   2. *S aureus*—older children and adults; 2nd most common cause
C. Classically involves a single joint, usually the knee
D. Presents as a warm joint with limited range of motion; fever, increased white count, and elevated ESR are often present.

VI. GOUT

[handwritten: → activate neutrophils]

A. Deposition of monosodium urate (MSU) crystals in tissues, especially the joints
B. Due to hyperuricemia; related to overproduction or decreased excretion of uric acid
   1. Uric acid is derived from purine metabolism and is excreted by the kidney.
C. Primary gout is the most common form; etiology of hyperuricemia is unknown.
D. Secondary gout is seen with *[handwritten: known cause]*
   1. Leukemia and myeloproliferative disorders—Increased cell turnover leads to hyperuricemia. *[handwritten: (tumor lysis syndrome)]*
   2. Lesch-Nyhan syndrome—X-linked deficiency of hypoxanthine-guanine phosphoribosyltransferase (HGPRT); presents with mental retardation and self-mutilation
   3. Renal insufficiency—decreased renal excretion of uric acid
E. Acute gout presents as exquisitely painful arthritis of the great toe (podagra)
   1. MSU crystals deposit in the joint, triggering an acute inflammatory reaction.
   2. Alcohol or consumption of meat may precipitate arthritis.
F. Chronic gout leads to
   1. Development of tophi—white, chalky aggregates of uric acid crystals with fibrosis and giant cell reaction in the soft tissue and joints (Fig. 18.9A)
   2. Renal failure—Urate crystals may deposit in kidney tubules (urate nephropathy).

[handwritten diagram, right margin:
Purines
↓
Xanthine
↓ Xanthine oxidase   (Recycled)
Uric Acid   HGPRT

AMP   GMP
↓   ↓
hypoxanthine   guanine
↓   ↓
Xanthine]

G. Laboratory findings include hyperuricemia; synovial fluid shows needle-shaped crystals with negative birefringence under polarized light (Fig. 18.9B).

yellow

H. Pseudogout resembles gout clinically, but is due to deposition of calcium pyrophosphate dihydrate (CPPD); synovial fluid shows rhomboid-shaped crystals with weakly positive birefringence under polarized light.

blue

SKELETAL MUSCLE

I. **DERMATOMYOSITIS**
   A. Inflammatory disorder of the skin and skeletal muscle
   B. Unknown etiology; some cases are associated with carcinoma (e.g., gastric carcinoma).
   C. Clinical features   *→ can't comb hair/climb stairs*
      1. Bilateral proximal muscle weakness; distal involvement can develop late in disease.
      2. Rash of the upper eyelids (heliotrope rash); malar rash may also be seen.
      3. Red papules on the elbows, knuckles, and knees (Gottron papules)
   D. Laboratory findings
      1. Increased creatine kinase
      2. Positive ANA and anti-Jo-1 antibody
      3. Perimysial inflammation (CD4+ T cells) with perifascicular atrophy on biopsy (Fig. 18.10)   *← closer to skin*
   E. Treatment is corticosteroids.

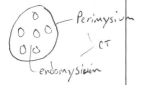

muscle fascicle

Perimysium

CT

endomysium

II. **POLYMYOSITIS**
   A. Inflammatory disorder of skeletal muscle
   B. Resembles dermatomyositis clinically, but skin is not involved; endomysial inflammation (CD8+ T cells) with necrotic muscle fibers is seen on biopsy.

III. **X-LINKED MUSCULAR DYSTROPHY**
   A. Degenerative disorder characterized by muscle wasting and replacement of skeletal muscle by adipose tissue
   B. Due to mutations of dystrophin
      1. Dystrophin is important for anchoring the muscle cytoskeleton to the extracellular matrix.
      2. Mutations are often spontaneous; large gene size predisposes to high rate of mutation.
   C. Duchenne muscular dystrophy is due to deletion of dystrophin.
      1. Presents as proximal muscle weakness at 1 year of age; progresses to involve distal muscles
         i. Calf pseudohypertrophy is a characteristic finding.
         ii. Serum creatine kinase is elevated.
      2. Death results from cardiac or respiratory failure; myocardium is commonly involved.
   D. Becker muscular dystrophy is due to mutated dystrophin; clinically results in milder disease   *→point mutation*

NEUROMUSCULAR JUNCTION

I. **MYASTHENIA GRAVIS**
   A. Autoantibodies against the postsynaptic acetylcholine receptor at the neuromuscular junction
   B. More commonly seen in women

C. Clinical features
 1. Muscle weakness that worsens with use and improves with rest; classically involves the eyes, leading to ptosis and diplopia
 2. Symptoms improve with anticholinesterase agents.
 3. Associated with thymic hyperplasia or thymoma; thymectomy improves symptoms.

II. LAMBERT-EATON SYNDROME
 A. Antibodies against presynaptic calcium channels of the neuromuscular junction
 B. Arises as a paraneoplastic syndrome, most commonly due to small cell carcinoma of the lung
 C. Leads to impaired acetylcholine release
 1. Firing of presynaptic calcium channels is required for acetylcholine release.
 D. Clinical features
 1. Proximal muscle weakness that improves with use; eyes are usually spared.
 2. Anticholinesterase agents do not improve symptoms.
 3. Resolves with resection of the cancer

SOFT TISSUE TUMORS

I. LIPOMA
 A. Benign tumor of adipose tissue
 B. Most common benign soft tissue tumor in adults

II. LIPOSARCOMA
 A. Malignant tumor of adipose tissue
 B. Most common malignant soft tissue tumor in adults
 C. Lipoblast is the characteristic cell.

III. RHABDOMYOMA
 A. Benign tumor of skeletal muscle
 B. Cardiac rhabdomyoma is associated with tuberous sclerosis.

IV. RHABDOMYOSARCOMA
 A. Malignant tumor of skeletal muscle
 B. Most common malignant soft tissue tumor in children
 C. Rhabdomyoblast is the characteristic cell; desmin positive
 D. Most common site is the head and neck; vagina is the classic site in young girls.

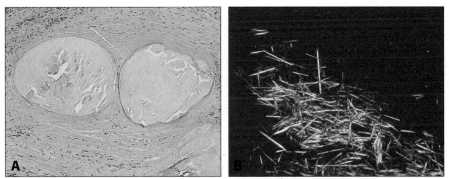

Fig. 18.9 Gout. **A**, Tophi. **B**, Negative birefringence. (B, Courtesy of Ed Uthman, MD)

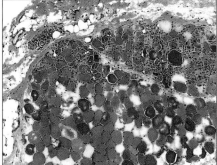

Fig. 18.10 Dermatomyositis. (Courtesy of Peter Pytel, MD)

Skin Pathology

19

INTRODUCTION

I. **SKIN**
   A. Functions as a barrier against environmental insults and fluid loss
   B. Composed of an epidermis and dermis separated by BM
   C. Epidermis is comprised of keratinocytes and has four layers (Fig. 19.1).
      1. Stratum basalis—regenerative (stem cell) layer
      2. Stratum spinosum—characterized by desmosomes between keratinocytes
      3. Stratum granulosum—characterized by granules in keratinocytes
      4. Stratum corneum—characterized by keratin in anucleate cells
   D. Dermis consists of connective tissue, nerve endings, blood and lymphatic vessels, and adnexal structures (e.g., hair shafts, sweat glands, and sebaceous glands).

INFLAMMATORY DERMATOSES

I. **ATOPIC (ECZEMATOUS) DERMATITIS**
   A. Pruritic, erythematous, oozing rash with vesicles and edema; often involves the face and flexor surfaces
   B. Type I hypersensitivity reaction; associated with asthma and allergic rhinitis

II. **CONTACT DERMATITIS**
   A. Pruritic, erythematous, oozing rash with vesicles and edema
   B. Arises upon exposure to allergens [Direct irritants] such as
      1. Poison ivy and nickel jewelry (type IV hypersensitivity)
      2. Irritant chemicals (e.g., detergents)
      3. Drugs (e.g., penicillin)
   C. Treatment involves removal of the offending agent and topical glucocorticoids, if needed.

III. **ACNE VULGARIS**   → scar of pustule
   A. Comedones (whiteheads and blackheads), pustules (pimples), and nodules; extremely common, especially in adolescents
   B. Due to chronic inflammation of hair follicles and associated sebaceous glands
      1. Hormone-associated increase in sebum production (sebaceous glands have androgen receptors) and excess keratin production block follicles, forming comedones.
      2. *Propionibacterium acnes* infection produces lipases that break down sebum, releasing proinflammatory fatty acids; results in pustule or nodule formation
   C. Treatment includes benzoyl peroxide (antimicrobial) and vitamin A derivatives (e.g., isotretinoin), which reduce keratin production.   ↳ maintain specialized epithelium

IV. **PSORIASIS**
   A. Well-circumscribed, salmon-colored plaques with silvery scale, usually on extensor surfaces and the scalp (Fig. 19.2A); pitting of nails may also be present.
   B. Due to excessive keratinocyte proliferation
                                    HLA-C

C. Possible autoimmune etiology
   1. Associated with HLA-C
   2. Lesions often arise in areas of trauma (environmental trigger).
D. Histology (Fig. 19.2B) shows
   1. Acanthosis (epidermal hyperplasia)
   2. Parakeratosis (hyperkeratosis with retention of keratinocyte nuclei in the stratum corneum)
   3. Collections of neutrophils in the stratum corneum (Munro microabscesses)
   4. Thinning of the epidermis above elongated dermal papillae; results in bleeding when scale is picked off (Auspitz sign)
E. Treatment involves corticosteroids, UV light with psoralen, or immune-modulating therapy.

(UV-A) → damage keratinocyte

V. LICHEN PLANUS

A. Pruritic, planar, polygonal, purple papules (Fig. 19.3A), often with reticular white lines on their surface (Wickham striae); commonly involves wrists, elbows, and oral mucosa
   1. Oral involvement manifests as Wickham striae.
B. Histology shows inflammation of the dermal-epidermal junction with a 'saw-tooth' appearance (Fig. 19.3B).
C. Etiology is unknown; associated with chronic hepatitis C virus infection

→ separation btwn layers

BLISTERING DERMATOSES

I. PEMPHIGUS VULGARIS

A. Autoimmune destruction of desmosomes between keratinocytes

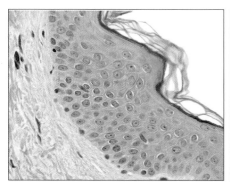

Fig. 19.1 Skin histology, normal.

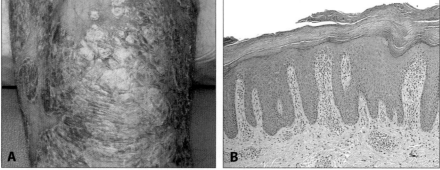

Fig. 19.2 Psoriasis. **A**, Clinical appearance. **B**, Microscopic appearance. (A, Courtesy of Vesna Petronic-Rosic, MD)

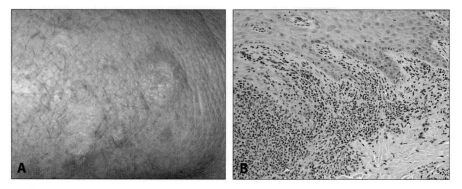

Fig. 19.3 Lichen planus. **A**, Clinical appearance. **B**, Microscopic appearance. (A, Courtesy of Vesna Petronic-Rosic, MD)

B. Due to IgG antibody against desmoglein (type II hypersensitivity)

C. Presents as skin and oral mucosa bullae (Fig. 19.4A).

   1. Acantholysis (separation) of stratum spinosum keratinocytes (normally connected by desmosomes) results in suprabasal blisters.

Seperation of keratinocyte

   2. Basal layer cells remain attached to basement membrane via hemidesmosomes ('tombstone' appearance, Fig. 19.4B).

   3. Thin-walled bullae rupture easily (Nikolsky sign), leading to shallow erosions with dried crust.

   4. Immunofluorescence highlights IgG surrounding keratinocytes in a 'fish net' pattern.

II. BULLOUS PEMPHIGOID

A. Autoimmune destruction of hemidesmosomes between basal cells and the underlying basement membrane

B. Due to IgG antibody against hemidesmosome components (BP180) of the basement membrane

C. Presents as blisters of the skin (Fig. 19.5A), usually in the elderly; oral mucosa is spared.

   1. Basal cell layer is detached from the basement membrane (Fig. 19.5B).

   2. Tense bullae do not rupture easily; clinically milder than pemphigus vulgaris

D. Immunofluorescence highlights IgG along basement membrane (linear pattern).

→ wall contains all of epidermis

III. DERMATITIS HERPETIFORMIS

A. Autoimmune deposition of IgA at the tips of dermal papillae

B. Presents as pruritic vesicles and bullae that are grouped (herpetiform, Fig. 19.6)

C. Strong association with celiac disease; resolves with gluten-free diet

blood vessels in dermal papillae

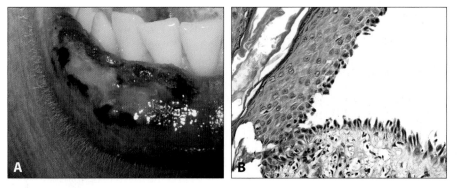

Fig. 19.4 Pemphigus vulgaris. **A**, Clinical appearance. **B**, Microscopic appearance. (A, Courtesy of Vesna Petronic-Rosic, MD)

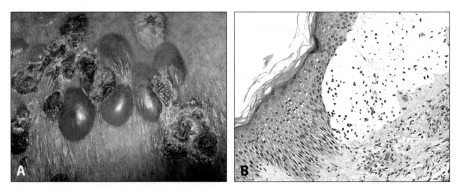

Fig. 19.5 Bullous pemphigoid. **A**, Clinical appearance. **B**, Microscopic appearance. (A, Courtesy of Vesna Petronic-Rosic, MD)

IV. **ERYTHEMA MULTIFORME (EM)**

   A. Hypersensitivity reaction characterized by targetoid rash and bullae (Fig. 19.7)

     1. Targetoid appearance is due to central epidermal necrosis surrounded by erythema.

   B. Most commonly associated with HSV infection; other associations include *Mycoplasma* infection, drugs (penicillin and sulfonamides), autoimmune disease (e.g., SLE), and malignancy.

   C. EM with oral mucosa/lip involvement and fever is termed Stevens-Johnson syndrome (SJS).

     1. Toxic epidermal necrolysis is a severe form of SJS characterized by diffuse sloughing of skin, resembling a large burn; most often due to an adverse drug reaction

EPITHELIAL TUMORS

I. **SEBORRHEIC KERATOSIS**

   A. Benign squamous proliferation; common tumor in the elderly

   B. Presents as raised, discolored plaques on the extremities or face; often has a coin-like, waxy, 'stuck-on' appearance (Fig. 19.8A)

     1. Characterized by keratin pseudocysts on histology (Fig. 19.8B)

   C. Leser-Trélat sign is the sudden onset of multiple seborrheic keratoses and suggests underlying carcinoma of the GI tract (Fig. 19.8C).

II. **ACANTHOSIS NIGRICANS**

   A. Epidermal hyperplasia with darkening of the skin ('velvet-like' skin, Fig. 19.9); often involves the axilla or groin

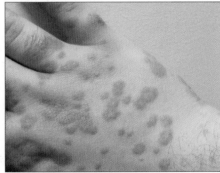

Fig. 19.6 Dermatitis herpetiformis. (Courtesy of Vesna Petronic-Rosic, MD)

Fig. 19.7 Erythema multiforme. (Courtesy of James Heilman, MD, Wikipedia)

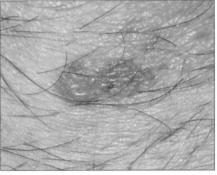

keratin pseudocyst

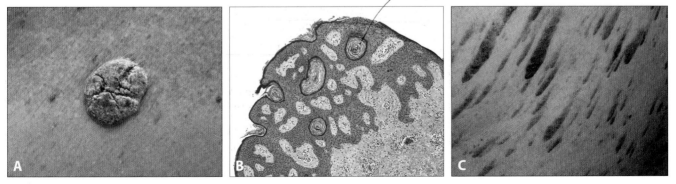

Fig. 19.8 Seborrheic keratosis. **A**, Clinical appearance. **B**, Microscopic appearance. **C**, Sign of Leser-Trélat. (A and C, Courtesy of Vesna Petronic-Rosic, MD)

B. Associated with insulin resistance (e.g., non-insulin-dependent diabetes) or malignancy (especially gastric carcinoma)

III. **BASAL CELL CARCINOMA**
   A. Malignant proliferation of the basal cells of the epidermis
      1. Most common cutaneous malignancy
   B. Risk factors stem from UVB-induced DNA damage and include prolonged exposure to sunlight, albinism, and xeroderma pigmentosum. →AR - no nucleotide excision repair - pyrimidine dimers
   C. Presents as an elevated nodule with a central, ulcerated crater surrounded by dilated (telangiectatic) vessels (Fig. 19.10A); 'pink, pearl-like papule'
      1. Classic location is the upper lip.
   D. Histology shows nodules of basal cells with peripheral palisading (Fig. 19.10B).
   E. Treatment is surgical excision; metastasis is rare.

IV. **SQUAMOUS CELL CARCINOMA**
   A. Malignant proliferation of squamous cells characterized by formation of keratin pearls.
   B. Risk factors stem from UVB-induced DNA damage and include prolonged exposure to sunlight, albinism, and xeroderma pigmentosum.
      1. Additional risk factors include immunosuppressive therapy, arsenic exposure, and chronic inflammation (e.g., scar from burn or draining sinus tract).
   C. Presents as an ulcerated, nodular mass, usually on the face (classically involving the lower lip)
   D. Treatment is excision; metastasis is uncommon.
   E. Actinic keratosis is a precursor lesion of squamous cell carcinoma and presents as a hyperkeratotic, scaly plaque, often on the face, back, or neck.
   F. Keratoacanthoma is well-differentiated squamous cell carcinoma that develops rapidly and regresses spontaneously; presents as a cup-shaped tumor filled with keratin debris

DISORDERS OF PIGMENTATION AND MELANOCYTES

I. **BASIC PRINCIPLES**
   A. Melanocytes are responsible for skin pigmentation and are present in the basal layer of the epidermis.
      1. Derived from the neural crest
      2. Synthesize melanin in melanosomes using tyrosine as a precursor molecule
      3. Pass melanosomes to keratinocytes

melanosomes └→tyrosine └→melanin └→passed to keratinocytes

Peripheral palisading

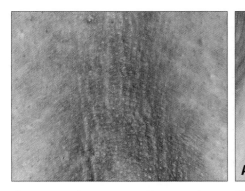
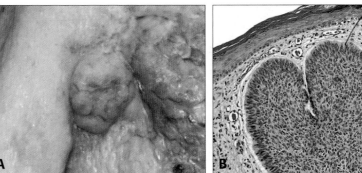

Fig. 19.9 Acanthosis nigricans. (Courtesy of Vesna Petronic-Rosic, MD)

Fig. 19.10 Basal cell carcinoma. **A**, Clinical appearance. **B**, Microscopic appearance. (A, Courtesy of Vesna Petronic-Rosic, MD)

II. **VITILIGO**
   A. Localized loss of skin pigmentation (Fig. 19.11)
   B. Due to autoimmune destruction of melanocytes

III. **ALBINISM**
   A. Congenital lack of pigmentation
   B. Due to an enzyme defect (usually tyrosinase) that impairs melanin production
   C. May involve the eyes (ocular form) or both the eyes and skin (oculocutaneous form)
   D. Increased risk of squamous cell carcinoma, basal cell carcinoma, and melanoma due to reduced protection against UVB

IV. **FRECKLE (EPHELIS)**
   A. Small, tan to brown macule; darkens when exposed to sunlight
   B. Due to increased number of melanosomes (melanocytes are not increased)

V. **MELASMA**
   A. Mask-like hyperpigmentation of the cheeks
   B. Associated with pregnancy and oral contraceptives

VI. **NEVUS (MOLE)**
   A. Benign neoplasm of melanocytes
   B. Congenital nevus is present at birth; often associated with hair (Fig. 19.12)
   C. Acquired nevus arises later in life.
      1. Begins as nests of melanocytes at the dermal-epidermal junction (junctional nevus); most common mole in children
      2. Grows by extension into the dermis (compound nevus)
      3. Junctional component is eventually lost resulting in an intradermal nevus, which is the most common mole in adults.
   D. Characterized by a flat macule or raised papule with symmetry, sharp borders, evenly distributed color, and small diameter (< 6 mm)
   E. Dysplasia may arise (dysplastic nevus), which is a precursor to melanoma.

VII. **MELANOMA** - no hair
   A. Malignant neoplasm of melanocytes; most common cause of death from skin cancer
   B. Risk factors are based on UVB-induced DNA damage and include prolonged exposure to sunlight, albinism, and xeroderma pigmentosum; an additional risk factor is dysplastic nevus syndrome (autosomal dominant disorder characterized by formation of dysplastic nevi that may progress to melanoma).
   C. Presents as a mole-like growth with "ABCD" (Fig. 19.13)

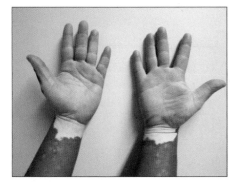

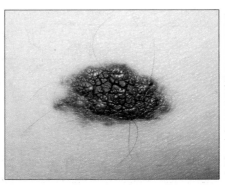

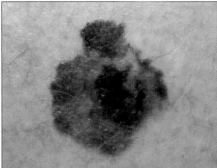

Fig. 19.11 Vitiligo. (Courtesy of James Heilman, MD, Wikipedia)

Fig. 19.12 Congenital nevus. (Courtesy of Vesna Petronic-Rosic, MD)

Fig. 19.13 Melanoma. (Courtesy of Vesna Petronic-Rosic, MD)

1. **A**symmetry
2. **B**orders are irregular.
3. **C**olor is not uniform.
4. **D**iameter > 6 mm

D. Characterized by two growth phases
   1. Radial growth horizontally along the epidermis and superficial dermis; low risk of metastasis
   2. Vertical growth into the deep dermis
      i. Increased risk of metastasis; depth of extension (Breslow thickness) is the most important prognostic factor in predicting metastasis.

E. Variants include
   1. Superficial spreading—most common subtype; dominant early radial growth results in good prognosis.
   2. Lentigo maligna melanoma—lentiginous proliferation (radial growth); good prognosis   *→ remain along dermal/epidermal junction*
   3. Nodular—early vertical growth; poor prognosis
   4. Acral lentiginous—arises on the palms or soles, often in dark-skinned individuals; not related to UV light exposure

[handwritten margin note: Grade
Breslow = vertical thickness
Clark = how deep it goes
(how many layers it penetrates)]

INFECTIOUS DISORDERS

I. **IMPETIGO**
   A. Superficial bacterial skin infection, most often due to *S aureus* or *S pyogenes*
   B. Commonly affects children
   C. Presents as erythematous macules that progress to pustules, usually on the face; *→ flat* rupture of pustules results in erosions and dry, crusted, honey-colored serum.

II. **CELLULITIS**
   A. Deeper (dermal and subcutaneous) infection, usually due to *S aureus* or *S pyogenes*
   B. Presents as a red, tender, swollen rash with fever
   C. Risk factors include recent surgery, trauma, or insect bite.
   D. Can progress to necrotizing fasciitis with necrosis of subcutaneous tissues due to infection with anaerobic 'flesh-eating' bacteria
      1. Production of CO_2 leads to crepitus.
      2. Surgical emergency

III. **STAPHYLOCOCCAL SCALDED SKIN SYNDROME**
   A. Sloughing of skin with erythematous rash and fever; leads to significant skin loss
   B. Due to *S aureus* infection; exfoliative A and B toxins result in epidermolysis of the stratum granulosum.

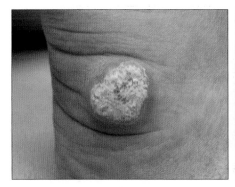

Fig. 19.14 Verruca. (Courtesy of Vesna Petronic-Rosic, MD)

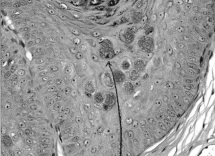

Fig. 19.15 Molluscum bodies. *filled w/ poxvirus*

C. Distinguished histologically from toxic epidermal necrolysis by level of skin separation; separation in TEN occurs at the dermal-epidermal junction.

IV. **VERRUCA (WART)**
   A. Flesh-colored papules with a rough surface (Fig. 19.14)
   B. Due to HPV infection of keratinocytes; characterized by koilocytic change
   C. Hands and feet are common locations.

V. **MOLLUSCUM CONTAGIOSUM**
   A. Firm, pink, umbilicated papules due to poxvirus; affected keratinocytes show cytoplasmic inclusions (molluscum bodies, Fig. 19.15)
   B. Most often arise in children; also occur in sexually active adults and immunocompromised individuals

Index